**Obstetrics and Gynecology Residency Match
Selection Criteria and Programs Requirements.**

By

**Match A Doc
and
Residency Guide**

Table of Contents

Obstetrics and Gynecology Residency Match Selection Criteria and Programs Requirements.

This book is the most single important piece you buy in your battle for residency. This is the **Obstetrics and Gynecology** Residency Match Selection Criteria and programs requirements book that contains up-to-date information about all the programs in the United States for both AMGs and IMGs. Why this book is essential to match? It has been shown that applying to programs that you don't match their minimum criteria is just waste of money and time. It is very important that you apply to those programs that you meet their requirements and this why we decided to make your life easier by gathering the information you need in one book. The information was gathered from program directors, coordinators, chiefs, faculty and residents. It includes Programs names, Programs codes, States, Addresses, Phones, Faxes, Percentage of IMGs in the programs, Minimum USMLE Step 1 and Step 2 Score Requirements, Attempts on any step, CS requirement at time of application, USCE Requirements, Cut-Off time since graduation, Programs offering couple match and Visas Sponsored or accepted. We have more than 10 years experience in the match field and our book is the proof that will help you to get the highest number of interviews to increase your chances in the match journey.

Alabama

University of South Alabama Obstetrics and Gynecology Residency Program

Specialty: Obstetrics and Gynecology OB GYN Residency
Program name: University of South Alabama Program
Program code: 220-01-21-020
NRMP Code: 1852220C0
Program type: University-based
State: Alabama
Address: University of South Alabama Medical Center,
          251 Cox St, Mobile, AL 36604
Phone: (251) 415-1557
Fax: (251) 415-1552
Percentage of IMGs in the program: 8%
Minimum USMLE Step 1 Score Requirement: No limits set
Minimum USMLE Step 2 Score Requirement: No limits set
Attempts on any step: Must pass on first attempt

CS required at time of application: Yes as well as ECFMG certificate
USCE Requirement: None
Cut-Off time since graduation: No limits set
Program offers couple match: Yes
Visas Sponsored or accepted: J1 visa

University of Alabama Medical Center Obstetrics and Gynecology Residency Program

Specialty: Obstetrics and Gynecology OB GYN Residency
Program name: University of Alabama Medical Center Program
Program code: 220-01-11-018
NRMP Code: 1007220C0
Program type: University-based
State: Alabama
Address: University of Alabama Medical Center, 619 19th St S, Birmingham, AL 35249-7333
Phone: (205) 934-5631
Fax: (205) 975-6411
Percentage of IMGs in the program: 0%
Minimum USMLE Step 1 Score Requirement: No limits set
Minimum USMLE Step 2 Score Requirement: No limits set
Attempts on any step: No limits set

CS required at time of application: Yes including ECFMG exam
USCE Requirement: None
Cut-Off time since graduation: No limits set
Program offers couple match: Yes
Visas Sponsored or accepted: J1 visa and H1b visa

Arizona

Banner Good Samaritan Medical Center Obstetrics and Gynecology Residency Program

Specialty: Obstetrics and Gynecology OB GYN Residency
Program name: Banner Good Samaritan Medical Center Program
Program code: 220-03-21-024
NRMP Code: 1011220C0
Program type: Community-based university affiliated hospital
State: Arizona
Address: Banner Good Samaritan Medical Center
1111 E McDowell Rd, Phoenix, AZ 85006-2666

Phone: (602) 839-3827
Fax: (602) 839-2359
Percentage of IMGs in the program: 0%
(occasionally 1 match)
Minimum USMLE Step 1 Score Requirement:
No limits set
Minimum USMLE Step 2 Score Requirement:
No limits set
Attempts on any step: No limits set
CS required at time of application: Yes as well
as ECFMG certificate
USCE Requirement: None
Cut-Off time since graduation: No limits set
Program offers couple match: Yes
Visas Sponsored or accepted: No visa

University of Arizona Obstetrics and Gynecology Residency Program

Specialty: Obstetrics and Gynecology OB GYN
Residency
Program name: University of Arizona Program
Program code: 220-03-21-025
NRMP Code: 1015220C0
Program type: University-based
State: Arizona
Address: University of Arizona Health Sciences
Center

        1501 N Campbell Ave, Tucson, AZ
85724

Phone: (520) 626-6636
Fax: (520) 626-1446
Percentage of IMGs in the program: 0%
Minimum USMLE Step 1 Score Requirement:
No limits set
Minimum USMLE Step 2 Score Requirement:
No limits set
Attempts on any step: No limits set
CS required at time of application: No
USCE Requirement: None
Cut-Off time since graduation: No limits set
Program offers couple match: Yes
Visas Sponsored or accepted: J1 visa

Phoenix Integrated Residency Obstetrics and Gynecology Residency Program

Specialty: Obstetrics and Gynecology OB GYN
Residency
Program name: Phoenix Integrated Residency
Program
Program code: 220-03-21-328
NRMP Code: 1898220C0, 1898220P0
Program type: Community-based university
affiliated hospital
State: Arizona
Address: Maricopa Medical Center
            2601 E Roosevelt St, Phoenix, AZ
85008

Phone: (602) 344-5084
Fax: (602) 344-5894
Percentage of IMGs in the program: 10%
Minimum USMLE Step 1 Score Requirement: 210
Minimum USMLE Step 2 Score Requirement: 210
Attempts on any step: Must pass maximum on 2nd attempt including CS exam
CS required at time of application: Yes including ECFMG certificate
USCE Requirement: None
Cut-Off time since graduation: No limits set
Program offers couple match: No
Visas Sponsored or accepted: No visa

Arkansas

University of Arkansas for Medical Sciences Obstetrics and Gynecology Residency Program

Specialty: Obstetrics and Gynecology OB GYN Residency
Program name: University of Arkansas for Medical Sciences Program

Program code: 220-04-11-026
NRMP Code: 1018220C0
Program type: University-based
State: Arkansas
Address: University of Arkansas for Medical Sciences

4301 W Markham St, Little Rock, AR 72205
Phone: (501) 526-7569
Fax: (501) 686-8945
Percentage of IMGs in the program: 0%
Minimum USMLE Step 1 Score Requirement: No limits set
Minimum USMLE Step 2 Score Requirement: No limits set
Attempts on any step: Must pass on the first attempt
CS required at time of application: No
USCE Requirement: None
Cut-Off time since graduation: 5 years
Program offers couple match: Yes
Visas Sponsored or accepted: J1 visa

California

University of Southern California/LAC+USC Medical Center Obstetrics and Gynecology Residency Program

Specialty: Obstetrics and Gynecology OB GYN Residency
Program name: University of Southern California/LAC+USC Medical Center Program
Program code: 220-05-11-036
NRMP Code: 1033220C0
Program type: University-based
State: California
Address: LAC+USC Medical Center
            1200 N State St, Los Angeles, CA 90033
Phone: (323) 409-8848
Percentage of IMGs in the program: 0%
Minimum USMLE Step 1 Score Requirement: No limits set
Minimum USMLE Step 2 Score Requirement: No limits set
Attempts on any step: No limits set
CS required at time of application: Yes including ECFMG certificate as well as PTAL/Status letter
USCE Requirement: None
Cut-Off time since graduation: No limits set
Program offers couple match: Yes
Visas Sponsored or accepted: J1 visa

Kaiser Permanente Southern California (Los Angeles) Obstetrics and Gynecology Residency Program

Specialty: Obstetrics and Gynecology OB GYN Residency
Program name: Kaiser Permanente Southern California (Los Angeles) Program
Program code: 220-05-12-035
State: California
Address: Kaiser Permanente Medical Center
393 E Walnut St, Pasadena, CA 91188
Phone: (877) 574-0002
Fax: (626) 405-6581
Percentage of IMGs in the program: 0%
Minimum USMLE Step 1 Score Requirement: No limits set
Minimum USMLE Step 2 Score Requirement: No limits set
Attempts on any step: No limits set
CS required at time of application: Yes including ECFMG certificate as well as PTAL/Status letter
USCE Requirement: None
Cut-Off time since graduation: No limits set
Program offers couple match: Yes
Visas Sponsored or accepted: No visa

Kaiser Permanente Medical Group (Northern California/Oakland) Obstetrics and Gynecology Residency Program

Specialty: Obstetrics and Gynecology OB GYN Residency

Program name: Kaiser Permanente Medical Group (Northern California/Oakland) Program

Program code: 220-05-12-040

NRMP Code: 1042220C0

Program type: Community-based university affiliated hospital

State: California

Address: Kaiser Permanente Oakland Medical Center

   3600 Broadway, Oakland, CA 94611

Phone: (510) 752-7772

Fax: (510) 752-1571

Percentage of IMGs in the program: 0%

Minimum USMLE Step 1 Score Requirement: 220

Minimum USMLE Step 2 Score Requirement: 220

Attempts on any step: No limits set

CS required at time of application: Yes including ECFMG certificate as well as PTAL/Status letter

USCE Requirement: None

Cut-Off time since graduation: No limits set

Program offers couple match: Yes
Visas Sponsored or accepted: No visa

Kaiser Permanente Medical Group (Northern California)/San Francisco Obstetrics and Gynecology Residency Program

Specialty: Obstetrics and Gynecology OB GYN Residency
Program name: Kaiser Permanente Medical Group (Northern California)/San Francisco Program
Program code: 220-05-12-045
NRMP Code: 1959220C0
Program type: Community-based
State: California
Address: Kaiser Permanente Medical Center
2425 Geary Blvd, San Francisco, CA 94115-3395
Phone: (415) 833-9183
Fax: (415) 833-4983
Percentage of IMGs in the program: 0%
Minimum USMLE Step 1 Score Requirement: No limits set
Minimum USMLE Step 2 Score Requirement: No limits set
Attempts on any step: No limits set

CS required at time of application: Yes including ECFMG certificate as well as PTAL/Status letter
USCE Requirement: None
Cut-Off time since graduation: No limits set
Program offers couple match: Yes
Visas Sponsored or accepted: No visa

Kaiser Permanente Medical Group (Northern California)/Santa Clara Obstetrics and Gynecology Residency Program

Specialty: Obstetrics and Gynecology OB GYN Residency
Program name: Kaiser Permanente Medical Group (Northern California)/Santa Clara Program
Program code: 220-05-12-311
State: California
Address: Kaiser Permanente Medical Center
710 Lawrence Expressway, Santa Clara, CA 95051-5386
Phone: (408) 851-3842
Fax: (408) 851-3839
Percentage of IMGs in the program: 0%
Minimum USMLE Step 1 Score Requirement: No limits set
Minimum USMLE Step 2 Score Requirement: No limits set

Attempts on any step: Must pass on first attempt including CS exam
CS required at time of application: Yes including ECFMG certificate as well as PTAL/Status letter
USCE Requirement: None
Cut-Off time since graduation: No limits set
Program offers couple match: Yes
Visas Sponsored or accepted: No visa

University of California (Davis) Health System Obstetrics and Gynecology Residency Program

Specialty: Obstetrics and Gynecology OB GYN Residency
Program name: University of California (Davis) Health System Program
Program code: 220-05-21-028
NRMP Code: 1046220C0
Program type: University-based
State: California
Address: UC Davis Medical Center
            4860 Y St, Sacramento, CA 95817
Phone: (916) 734-6978
Fax: (916) 734-6666
Percentage of IMGs in the program: 0%
Minimum USMLE Step 1 Score Requirement: No limits set

Minimum USMLE Step 2 Score Requirement:
No limits set
Attempts on any step: No limits set
CS required at time of application: No
but PTAL/Status letter required
USCE Requirement: None
Cut-Off time since graduation: 5 years
Program offers couple match: Yes
Visas Sponsored or accepted: J1 visa and H1b
visa

University of California (Irvine) Obstetrics and Gynecology Residency Program

Specialty: Obstetrics and Gynecology OB GYN
Residency
Program name: University of California (Irvine)
Program
Program code: 220-05-21-031
NRMP Code: 1043220C0
Program type: University-based
State: California
Address: UC Irvine Medical Center
          101 The City Dr S, Orange, CA 92868
Phone: (714) 456-8224
Fax: (714) 456-8360
Percentage of IMGs in the program: 0%
Minimum USMLE Step 1 Score Requirement:
210

Minimum USMLE Step 2 Score Requirement:
210
Attempts on any step: Must pass on first attempt
CS required at time of application: Yes including ECFMG certificate as well as PTAL/Status letter
USCE Requirement: Yes
Cut-Off time since graduation: No limits set
Program offers couple match: Yes
Visas Sponsored or accepted: J1 visa

White Memorial Medical Center Obstetrics and Gynecology Residency Program

Specialty: Obstetrics and Gynecology OB GYN Residency
Program name: White Memorial Medical Center Program
Program code: 220-05-21-039
NRMP Code: 1040220C0
Program type: Community-based university affiliated hospital
State: California
Address: White Memorial Medical Center
1720 Cesar E Chavez Ave, Los Angeles, CA 90033
Phone: (323) 260-5810

Fax: (323) 881-8601
Percentage of IMGs in the program: 0%
Minimum USMLE Step 1 Score Requirement: No limits set
Minimum USMLE Step 2 Score Requirement: No limits set
Attempts on any step: No limits set
CS required at time of application: Yes including ECFMG certificate as well as PTAL/Status letter
USCE Requirement: None
Cut-Off time since graduation: No limits set
Program offers couple match: Yes
Visas Sponsored or accepted: J1 visa

University of California (San Diego) Obstetrics and Gynecology Residency Program

Specialty: Obstetrics and Gynecology OB GYN Residency
Program name: University of California (San Diego) Program
Program code: 220-05-21-044
NRMP Code: 1049220C0
Program type: University-based
State: California
Address: UCSD Medical Center
          200 W Arbor Dr, San Diego, CA 92103-8433

Phone: (619) 543-6922
Fax: (619) 543-5767
Percentage of IMGs in the program: 0%
Minimum USMLE Step 1 Score Requirement: No limits set
Minimum USMLE Step 2 Score Requirement: No limits set
Attempts on any step: Must pass on first attempt including CS exam
CS required at time of application: No but PTAL/Status letter required
USCE Requirement: None
Cut-Off time since graduation: No limits set
Program offers couple match: Yes
Visas Sponsored or accepted: No visa

University of California (San Francisco) Obstetrics and Gynecology Residency Program

Specialty: Obstetrics and Gynecology OB GYN Residency
Program name: University of California (San Francisco) Program
Program code: 220-05-21-047
State: California
Address: San Francisco General Hospital 1001 Potrero Ave, San Francisco, CA 94110
Phone: (415) 206-3061

Fax: (415) 206-3112
Percentage of IMGs in the program: 0%
**Minimum USMLE Step 1 Score
Requirement:** No limits set
**Minimum USMLE Step 2 Score
Requirement:** No limits set
Attempts on any step: Must pass on first
attempt
CS required at time of application: No
but PTAL/Status letter is required
USCE Requirement: None
Cut-Off time since graduation: No limits
set
Program offers couple match: No
Visas Sponsored or accepted: J1 visa and
H1b visa

Stanford University Obstetrics and Gynecology Residency Program

Specialty: Obstetrics and Gynecology OB GYN
Residency
Program name: Stanford University Program
Program code: 220-05-21-048
State: California
Address: Stanford University Medical Center
          300 Pasteur Dr, Stanford, CA 94305-
5317
Phone: (650) 498-7570

Fax: (650) 723-7737
Percentage of IMGs in the program: 0%
Minimum USMLE Step 1 Score Requirement: No limits set
Minimum USMLE Step 2 Score Requirement: No limits set
Attempts on any step: Must pass on first attempt
CS required at time of application: No but PTAL/Status letter is required
USCE Requirement: None
Cut-Off time since graduation: No limits set
Program offers couple match: Yes
Visas Sponsored or accepted: No visa

Los Angeles County-Harbor-UCLA Medical Center Obstetrics and Gynecology Residency Program

Specialty: Obstetrics and Gynecology OB GYN Residency
Program name: Los Angeles County-Harbor-UCLA Medical Center Program
Program code: 220-05-21-050
State: California
Address: Los Angeles County-Harbor-UCLA Medical Center
        1000 W Carson St, Torrance, CA 90509
Phone: (310) 222-3886
Fax: (310) 782-8148

Percentage of IMGs in the program: 0%
Minimum USMLE Step 1 Score Requirement: 200
Minimum USMLE Step 2 Score Requirement: 210
Attempts on any step: Must pass on first attempt including CS exam
CS required at time of application: Yes including ECFMG certificate as well as PTAL/Status letter
USCE Requirement: None
Cut-Off time since graduation: 2 years
Program offers couple match: Yes
Visas Sponsored or accepted: No visa

Loma Linda University Obstetrics and Gynecology Residency Program

Specialty: Obstetrics and Gynecology OB GYN Residency
Program name: Loma Linda University Program
Program code: 220-05-21-329
State: California
Address: Loma Linda University Medical Center
        11234 Anderson St, Loma Linda, CA 92354
Phone: (909) 651-5534
Fax: (909) 651-5401
Percentage of IMGs in the program: 10%

Minimum USMLE Step 1 Score Requirement:
No limits set
Minimum USMLE Step 2 Score Requirement:
No limits set
Attempts on any step: No limits set
CS required at time of application: No
but PTAL/Status letter is required
USCE Requirement: None
Cut-Off time since graduation: 5 years
Program offers couple match: Yes
Visas Sponsored or accepted: J1 visa

Santa Clara Valley Medical Center Obstetrics and Gynecology Residency Program

Specialty: Obstetrics and Gynecology OB GYN
Residency
Program name: Santa Clara Valley Medical
Center Program
Program code: 220-05-21-333
NRMP Code: 1063220C0
Program type: Community-based
State: California
Address: Santa Clara Valley Medical Center
          751 S Bascom Ave, San Jose, CA 95128
Phone: (408) 885-5550
Fax: (408) 885-5577
Percentage of IMGs in the program: 0%

Minimum USMLE Step 1 Score Requirement:
No limits set
Minimum USMLE Step 2 Score Requirement:
No limits set
Attempts on any step: No limits set
CS required at time of application: No
but PTAL/Status letter is required
USCE Requirement: None
Cut-Off time since graduation: No limits set
Program offers couple match: Yes
Visas Sponsored or accepted: No visa

Kern Medical Center Obstetrics and Gynecology Residency Program

Specialty: Obstetrics and Gynecology OB GYN Residency
Program name: Kern Medical Center Program
Program code: 220-05-31-027
NRMP Code: 1921220C0
Program type: Community-based
State: California
Address: Kern Medical Center
1700 Mount Vernon Ave,
Bakersfield, CA 93306
Phone: (661) 326-2237
Fax: (661) 326-2235
Percentage of IMGs in the program: 10% (variable)

Minimum USMLE Step 1 Score Requirement: No limits set
Minimum USMLE Step 2 Score Requirement: No limits set
Attempts on any step: Must pass on first attempt
CS required at time of application: Yes including ECFMG certificate as well as PTAL/Status letter
USCE Requirement: None
Cut-Off time since graduation: No limits set
Program offers couple match: Yes
Visas Sponsored or accepted: No visa

University of California (San Francisco)/Fresno Obstetrics and Gynecology Residency Program

Specialty: Obstetrics and Gynecology OB GYN Residency
Program name: University of California (San Francisco)/Fresno Program
Program code: 220-05-31-029
NRMP Code: 1022220C0
Program type: Community-based university affiliated hospital
State: California

Address: UCSF Fresno
           155 N Fresno St, Fresno, CA 93701
Phone: (559) 499-6545
Fax: (559) 499-6541
Percentage of IMGs in the program: 0%
Minimum USMLE Step 1 Score Requirement: No limits set
Minimum USMLE Step 2 Score Requirement: No limits set
Attempts on any step: Must pass on first attempt
CS required at time of application: No but PTAL/Status letter is required
USCE Requirement: None
Cut-Off time since graduation: No limits set
Program offers couple match: Yes
Visas Sponsored or accepted: J1 visa

UCLA Medical Center Obstetrics and Gynecology Residency Program

Specialty: Obstetrics and Gynecology OB GYN Residency
Program name: UCLA Medical Center Program
Program code: 220-05-31-038
NRMP Code: 1956220P0, 1956220C0
Program type: University-based
State: California

Address: UCLA Medical Center
        10833 Le Conte Ave, Los Angeles, CA 90095-1740
Phone: (310) 825-9945
Fax: (310) 206-7186
Percentage of IMGs in the program: 5%
Minimum USMLE Step 1 Score Requirement: No limits set
Minimum USMLE Step 2 Score Requirement: No limits set
Attempts on any step: Must pass maximum from 2nd attempt
CS required at time of application: Yes including ECFMG certificate as well as PTAL/Status letter
USCE Requirement: None
Cut-Off time since graduation: No limits set
Program offers couple match: Yes
Visas Sponsored or accepted: J1 visa

Cedars-Sinai Medical Center Obstetrics and Gynecology Residency Program

Specialty: Obstetrics and Gynecology OB GYN Residency
Program name: Cedars-Sinai Medical Center Program
Program code: 220-05-31-034

NRMP Code: 1030220C0
Program type: Community-based university affiliated hospital
State: California
Address: Cedars-Sinai Medical Center
          8700 Beverly Blvd, Los Angeles, CA 90048
Phone: (310) 423-7417
Fax: (310) 423-0313
Percentage of IMGs in the program: 0%
Minimum USMLE Step 1 Score Requirement: No limits set
Minimum USMLE Step 2 Score Requirement: No limits set
Attempts on any step: No limits set
CS required at time of application: Yes including ECFMG certificate as well as PTAL/Status letter
USCE Requirement: Yes
Cut-Off time since graduation: No limits set
Program offers couple match: Yes
Visas Sponsored or accepted: J1 visa and H1b visa

Colorado

Exempla St Joseph Hospital Obstetrics and Gynecology Residency Program

Specialty: Obstetrics and Gynecology OB GYN Residency
Program name: Exempla St Joseph Hospital Program
Program code: 220-07-21-051
NRMP Code: 1074220C0
Program type: Community-based
State: Colorado
Address: St Joseph Hospital
1960 Ogden St, Denver, CO 80218-1191
Phone: (303) 318-3270
Fax: (303) 318-3274
Percentage of IMGs in the program: 0%
Minimum USMLE Step 1 Score Requirement: 210
Minimum USMLE Step 2 Score Requirement: 215
Attempts on any step: Must pass on first attempt
CS required at time of application: Yes
USCE Requirement: Yes
Cut-Off time since graduation: 3 years
Program offers couple match: Yes
Visas Sponsored or accepted: No visa

University of Colorado Obstetrics and Gynecology Residency Program

Specialty: Obstetrics and Gynecology OB GYN Residency
Program name: University of Colorado Program
Program code: 220-07-31-052
NRMP Code: 1076220P0, 1076220C0
Program type: University-based
State: Colorado
Address: University of Colorado Denver School of Medicine

      12631 E 17th Ave, Aurora, CO 80045
Phone: (303) 724-2052
Fax: (303) 724-2055
Percentage of IMGs in the program: 8%
Minimum USMLE Step 1 Score Requirement: 220
Minimum USMLE Step 2 Score Requirement: 220
Attempts on any step: Must pass on first attempt including CS exam
CS required at time of application: Yes including ECFMG certificate
USCE Requirement: None
Cut-Off time since graduation: No limits set
Program offers couple match: Yes
Visas Sponsored or accepted: J1 visa

Connecticut

Bridgeport Hospital/Yale University Obstetrics and Gynecology Residency Program

Specialty: Obstetrics and Gynecology OB GYN Residency
Program name: Bridgeport Hospital/Yale University Program
Program code: 220-08-11-054
NRMP Code: 1079220C0
Program type: Community-based university affiliated hospital
State: Connecticut
Address: Bridgeport Hospital
          267 Grant St, Bridgeport, CT 06610
Phone: (203) 384-3990
Fax: (203) 384-3715
Percentage of IMGs in the program: 40%
Minimum USMLE Step 1 Score Requirement: No limits set
Minimum USMLE Step 2 Score Requirement: No limits set
Attempts on any step: No limits set
CS required at time of application: No
USCE Requirement: None
Cut-Off time since graduation: No limits set
Program offers couple match: Yes

Visas Sponsored or accepted: J1 visa and H1b visa

St Francis Hospital and Medical Center Obstetrics and Gynecology Residency Program

Specialty: Obstetrics and Gynecology OB GYN Residency
Program name: St Francis Hospital and Medical Center Program
Program code: 220-08-11-059
State: Connecticut
Address: St Francis Hospital and Medical Center
114 Woodland St, Hartford, CT 06105
Phone: (860) 714-5170
Fax: (860) 714-8008
Percentage of IMGs in the program: 0%
Minimum USMLE Step 1 Score Requirement: No limits set
Minimum USMLE Step 2 Score Requirement: No limits set
Attempts on any step: Must pass on first attempt including CS exam
CS required at time of application: No
USCE Requirement: None
Cut-Off time since graduation: No limits set
Program offers couple match: No
Visas Sponsored or accepted: J1 visa

Stamford Hospital/Columbia University College of Physicians and Surgeons Obstetrics and Gynecology Residency Program

Specialty: Obstetrics and Gynecology OB GYN Residency
Program name: Stamford Hospital/Columbia University College of Physicians and Surgeons Program
Program code: 220-08-11-061
NRMP Code: 1095220C0
Program type: Community-based university affiliated hospital
State: Connecticut
Address: Stamford Hospital
　　　　　30 Shelburne Rd, Stamford, CT 06904
Phone: (203) 276-7581
Fax: (203) 276-7259
Percentage of IMGs in the program: 0%
Minimum USMLE Step 1 Score Requirement: No limits set
Minimum USMLE Step 2 Score Requirement: No limits set
Attempts on any step: No limits set
CS required at time of application: Yes including ECFMG certificate
USCE Requirement: Yes
Cut-Off time since graduation: 5 years
Program offers couple match: Yes

Visas Sponsored or accepted: No visa

Danbury Hospital Obstetrics and Gynecology Residency Program

Specialty: Obstetrics and Gynecology OB GYN Residency
Program name: Danbury Hospital Program
Program code: 220-08-21-055
NRMP Code: 1081220C0
Program type: Community-based university affiliated hospital
State: Connecticut
Address: Danbury Hospital
        24 Hospital Ave, Danbury, CT 06810
Phone: (203) 739-7872
Fax: (203) 739-8694
Percentage of IMGs in the program: 0%
Minimum USMLE Step 1 Score Requirement: No limits set
Minimum USMLE Step 2 Score Requirement: No limits set
Attempts on any step: No limits set
CS required at time of application: Yes
USCE Requirement: None
Cut-Off time since graduation: 2 years
Program offers couple match: Yes
Visas Sponsored or accepted: J1 visa and H1b visa

Yale-New Haven Medical Center Obstetrics and Gynecology Residency Program

Specialty: Obstetrics and Gynecology OB GYN Residency
Program name: Yale-New Haven Medical Center Program
Program code: 220-08-21-060
NRMP Code: 1089220C0, 1089220P1
Program type: University-based
State: Connecticut
Address: Yale-New Haven Medical Center
             333 Cedar St, New Haven, CT 06520-8063
Phone: (203) 785-4004
Fax: (203) 785-6586
Percentage of IMGs in the program: 0% (Occasional 1)
Minimum USMLE Step 1 Score Requirement: 215
Minimum USMLE Step 2 Score Requirement: No limits set
Attempts on any step: No limits set
CS required at time of application: No
USCE Requirement: Yes 1 month
Cut-Off time since graduation: No limits set
Program offers couple match: Yes
Visas Sponsored or accepted: J1 visa (H1b visa for exceptional candidates)

University of Connecticut Obstetrics and Gynecology Residency Program

Specialty: Obstetrics and Gynecology OB GYN Residency
Program name: University of Connecticut Program
Program code: 220-08-21-355
NRMP Code: 1094220C0
Program type: Community-based university affiliated hospital
State: Connecticut
Address: University of Connecticut Health Center
          263 Farmington Ave, Farmington, CT 06030-2947
Phone: (860) 679-2853
Fax: (860) 679-1228
Percentage of IMGs in the program: 0%
Minimum USMLE Step 1 Score Requirement: No limits set
Minimum USMLE Step 2 Score Requirement: No limits set
Attempts on any step: Must pass on first attempt including CS exam
CS required at time of application: Yes including ECFMG certificate
USCE Requirement: None
Cut-Off time since graduation: No limits set

Program offers couple match: Yes
Visas Sponsored or accepted: J1 visa

Delaware

Christiana Care Health Services Obstetrics and Gynecology Residency Program

Specialty: Obstetrics and Gynecology OB GYN Residency
Program name: Christiana Care Health Services Program
Program code: 220-09-11-062
NRMP Code: 1099220C0
Program type: Community-based university affiliated hospital
State: Delaware
Address: Christiana Care Health System
          4755 Ogletown-Stanton Rd, Newark, DE 19713
Phone: (302) 733-6565
Fax: (302) 733-2330
Percentage of IMGs in the program: 0%
Minimum USMLE Step 1 Score Requirement: 210

Minimum USMLE Step 2 Score Requirement: 210
Attempts on any step: Must pass on first attempt including CS exam
CS required at time of application: Yes including ECFMG certificate
USCE Requirement: None
Cut-Off time since graduation: No limits set
Program offers couple match: Yes
Visas Sponsored or accepted: J1 visa

District of Columbia

Washington Hospital Center Obstetrics and Gynecology Residency Program

Specialty: Obstetrics and Gynecology
Program name: Washington Hospital Center Program
Program code: 220-10-31-067
NRMP Code: 1800220C0
Program type: Community-based University affiliated hospital
State: District of Columbia

Address: Washington Hospital Center
110 Irving St NW, Washington, DC 20010-2975
Phone: (202) 877-8035
Fax: (202) 877-5435
Percentage of IMGs in the program: 10%
Minimum USMLE Step 1 Score Requirement: No limits set
Minimum USMLE Step 2 Score Requirement: No limits set
Attempts on any step: No limits set
CS required at time of application: Yes
USCE Requirement: None
Cut-Off time since graduation: No limits set
Program offers couple match: Yes
Visas Sponsored or accepted: J1 visa

Howard University Obstetrics and Gynecology Residency Program

Specialty: Obstetrics and Gynecology
Program name: Howard University Program
Program code: 220-10-21-065
State: District of Columbia
Address: Howard University Hospital
2041 Georgia Ave NW, Washington, DC 20060
Phone: (202) 865-7081
Fax: (202) 865-4165
Percentage of IMGs in the program: 0%

Minimum USMLE Step 1 Score Requirement: No limits set
Minimum USMLE Step 2 Score Requirement: No limits set
Attempts on any step: Must pass on first attempt including CS exam
CS required at time of application: Yes including ECFMG certificate
USCE Requirement: None
Cut-Off time since graduation: No limits set
Program offers couple match: No
Visas Sponsored or accepted: J1 visa and H1b visa

George Washington University Obstetrics and Gynecology Residency Program

Specialty: Obstetrics and Gynecology
Program name: George Washington University Program
Program code: 220-10-21-064
State: District of Columbia
Address: George Washington University Medical Center
          2150 Pennsylvania Ave NW, Washington, DC 20037
Phone: (202) 741-2532
Fax: (202) 741-2550
Percentage of IMGs in the program: 10%

Minimum USMLE Step 1 Score Requirement: 220
Minimum USMLE Step 2 Score Requirement: 220
Attempts on any step: Must pass on first attempt
CS required at time of application: No
USCE Requirement: None
Cut-Off time since graduation: No limits set
Program offers couple match: Yes
Visas Sponsored or accepted: J1 visa

Florida

University of Florida Obstetrics and Gynecology Residency Program

Specialty: Obstetrics and Gynecology
Program name: University of Florida Program
Program code: 220-11-11-068
NRMP Code: 1824220C0
Program type: University-based
State: Florida
Address: University of Florida College of Medicine
        1600 SW Archer Rd, Gainesville, FL 32610-0294

Phone:(352) 273-7943
Fax:(352) 294-5096
Percentage of IMGs in the program: 0%
Minimum USMLE Step 1 Score Requirement: 225
Minimum USMLE Step 2 Score Requirement: 225
Attempts on any step: Must pass on first attempt including CS exam
CS required at time of application: Yes including ECFMG certificate
USCE Requirement: None
Cut-Off time since graduation: No limits set
Program offers couple match: Yes
Visas Sponsored or accepted: J1 visa

Bayfront Medical Center Obstetrics and Gynecology Residency Program

Specialty: Obstetrics and Gynecology
Program name: Bayfront Medical Center Program
Program code: 220-11-11-074
NRMP Code: 1911220C0
Program type: Community-based
State: Florida
Address: Bayfront Health St Petersburg
700 6th St S, St Petersburg, FL 33701
Phone: (727) 893-6917

Fax: (727) 893-6978
Percentage of IMGs in the program: 40%
Minimum USMLE Step 1 Score Requirement:
No limits set
Minimum USMLE Step 2 Score Requirement:
No limits set
Attempts on any step: No limits set
CS required at time of application: Yes
including ECFMG certificate
USCE Requirement: None
Cut-Off time since graduation: No limits set
Program offers couple match: Yes
Visas Sponsored or accepted: No visa

Orlando Health Obstetrics and Gynecology Residency Program

Specialty: Obstetrics and Gynecology
Program name: Orlando Health Program
Program code: 220-11-12-072
State: Florida
Address: Orlando Health
          1401 Lucerne Terrace, Orlando, FL
32806-2093
Phone: (407) 841-5297
Fax: (407) 481-0182
Percentage of IMGs in the program: 0%
Minimum USMLE Step 1 Score Requirement:
No limits set

Minimum USMLE Step 2 Score Requirement: No limits set
Attempts on any step: Must pass on first attempt including CS exam
CS required at time of application: Yes including ECFMG certificate
USCE Requirement: None but if YOG > 3 years then 1 year USCE required
Cut-Off time since graduation: 3 years, if more then 1 year USCE is required
Program offers couple match: Yes
Visas Sponsored or accepted: No visa

University of Florida College of Medicine Jacksonville Obstetrics and Gynecology Residency Program

Specialty: Obstetrics and Gynecology
Program name: University of Florida College of Medicine Jacksonville Program
Program code: 220-11-21-069
NRMP Code: 1101220C0
Program type: Community-based university affiliated hospital
State: Florida
Address: University of Florida College of Medicine Jacksonville
        653-1 W 8th St, Jacksonville, FL 32209
Phone: (904) 244-3112

Fax: (904) 244-3658
Percentage of IMGs in the program: 0%
Minimum USMLE Step 1 Score Requirement: 200
Minimum USMLE Step 2 Score Requirement: 205
Attempts on any step: No limits set
CS required at time of application: Yes including ECFMG certificate
USCE Requirement: None
Cut-Off time since graduation: No limits set
Program offers couple match: Yes
Visas Sponsored or accepted: J1 visa and H1b visa

Jackson Memorial Hospital/Jackson Health System Obstetrics and Gynecology Residency Program

Specialty: Obstetrics and Gynecology
Program name: Jackson Memorial Hospital/Jackson Health System Program
Program code: 220-11-21-070
NRMP Code: 1104220C0
Program type: University-based
State: Florida
Address: University of Miami/Jackson Memorial Hospital
      1161 NW 12th Ave, Miami, FL 33136
Phone: (305) 585-5640

Fax: (305) 585-7651
Percentage of IMGs in the program: 30%
Minimum USMLE Step 1 Score Requirement: 220
Minimum USMLE Step 2 Score Requirement: 220
Attempts on any step: Must pass maximum on 2nd attempt including CS exam
CS required at time of application: No
USCE Requirement: None
Cut-Off time since graduation: 10 years
Program offers couple match: Yes
Visas Sponsored or accepted: J1 visa

Florida State University College of Medicine (Pensacola) Obstetrics and Gynecology Residency Program

Specialty: Obstetrics and Gynecology
Program name: Florida State University College of Medicine (Pensacola) Program
Program code: 220-11-21-073
NRMP Code: 1826220C0
Program type: Community-based university affiliated hospital
State: Florida
Address: Florida State University College of Medicine
          5045 Carpenter Creek Dr, Pensacola, FL 32503

Phone: (850) 416-2418
Fax: (850) 416-2460
Percentage of IMGs in the program: 0%
Minimum USMLE Step 1 Score Requirement: 200
Minimum USMLE Step 2 Score Requirement: 220
Attempts on any step: No limits set
CS required at time of application: Yes including ECFMG certificate
USCE Requirement: None
Cut-Off time since graduation: No limits set
Program offers couple match: Yes
Visas Sponsored or accepted: No visa

University of South Florida Morsani Obstetrics and Gynecology Residency Program

Specialty: Obstetrics and Gynecology
Program name: University of South Florida Morsani Program
Program code: 220-11-21-075
NRMP Code: 1109220C0
Program type: University-based
State: Florida
Address: USF Health Tampa General Hospital
            2 Tampa General Circle, Tampa, FL 33606
Phone: (813) 259-8876

Fax: (813) 250-2560
Percentage of IMGs in the program: 0%
Minimum USMLE Step 1 Score Requirement: No limits set
Minimum USMLE Step 2 Score Requirement: No limits set
Attempts on any step: Must pass on first attempt
CS required at time of application: Yes including ECFMG certificate
USCE Requirement: None
Cut-Off time since graduation: No limits set
Program offers couple match: Yes
Visas Sponsored or accepted: J1 visa

Georgia

Medical Center of Central Georgia/Mercer University School of Medicine Obstetrics and Gynecology Residency Program

Specialty: Obstetrics and Gynecology
Program name: Medical Center of Central Georgia/Mercer University School of Medicine Program
Program code: 220-12-11-079

State: Georgia
Address: Medical Center of Central Georgia
729 Pine St, Macon, GA 31201
Phone: (478) 633-1056
Percentage of IMGs in the program: 50%
Minimum USMLE Step 1 Score Requirement:
No limits set
Minimum USMLE Step 2 Score Requirement:
No limits set
Attempts on any step: No limits set
CS required at time of application: Yes
USCE Requirement: None
Cut-Off time since graduation: 10 years
Program offers couple match: Yes
Visas Sponsored or accepted: No visa

Memorial Health-University Medical Center/Mercer University School of Medicine (Savannah) Obstetrics and Gynecology Residency Program

Specialty: Obstetrics and Gynecology
Program name: Memorial Health-University
Medical Center/Mercer University School of
Medicine (Savannah) Program
Program code: 220-12-11-080
NRMP Code: 1971220C0
Program type: Community-based university

affiliated hospital
State: Georgia
Address: Memorial University Medical Center
        4700 Waters Ave, Savannah, GA 31404
Phone: (912) 350-3595
Fax: (912) 350-7969
Percentage of IMGs in the program: 0%
Minimum USMLE Step 1 Score Requirement:
200
Minimum USMLE Step 2 Score Requirement:
210
Attempts on any step: Must pass on first
attempt including CS exam
CS required at time of application: No
USCE Requirement: Yes
Cut-Off time since graduation: No limits set
Program offers couple match: Yes
Visas Sponsored or accepted: No visa

Emory University Obstetrics and Gynecology Residency Program

Specialty: Obstetrics and Gynecology
Program name: Emory University Program
Program code: 220-12-21-076
NRMP Code: 1113220C0
Program type: University-based
State: Georgia
Address: Grady Memorial Hospital
        69 Jesse Hill Jr Dr SE, Atlanta, GA

30303
Phone: (404) 251-8800
Fax: (404) 521-3589
Percentage of IMGs in the program: 0%
(Occasionally one)
Minimum USMLE Step 1 Score Requirement:
200
Minimum USMLE Step 2 Score Requirement:
210
Attempts on any step: Must pass on first
attempt
CS required at time of application: Yes
including ECFMG certificate
USCE Requirement: Yes
Cut-Off time since graduation: 5 years
Program offers couple match: Yes
Visas Sponsored or accepted: J1 visa and H1b
visa

Medical College of Georgia Obstetrics and Gynecology Residency Program

Specialty: Obstetrics and Gynecology
Program name: Medical College of Georgia
Program
Program code: 220-12-21-078
NRMP Code: 1985220C0
State: Georgia

Address: Georgia Regents University MCG
          1120 15th St, Augusta, GA 30912-3305
Phone: (706) 721-2541
Fax: (706) 721-2122
Percentage of IMGs in the program: 10%
Minimum USMLE Step 1 Score Requirement: 200
Minimum USMLE Step 2 Score Requirement: 210
Attempts on any step: Must pass maximum on the 2nd attempt including CS exam
CS required at time of application: Yes including ECFMG certificate
USCE Requirement: Yes
Cut-Off time since graduation: 2 years
Program offers couple match: Yes
Visas Sponsored or accepted: J1 visa

Morehouse School of Medicine Obstetrics and Gynecology Residency Program

Specialty: Obstetrics and Gynecology
Program name: Morehouse School of Medicine Program
Program code: 220-12-21-348
NRMP Code: 2099220C0
Program type: University-based
State: Georgia

Address: Morehouse School of Medicine
720 Westview Dr SW, Atlanta, GA 30310-1495
Phone: (404) 616-1692
Fax: (404) 616-4131
Percentage of IMGs in the program: 0% (Occasionally one)
Minimum USMLE Step 1 Score Requirement: No limits set
Minimum USMLE Step 2 Score Requirement: No limits set
Attempts on any step: No limits set
CS required at time of application: Yes including ECFMG certificate
USCE Requirement: Yes
Cut-Off time since graduation: No limits set
Program offers couple match: No
Visas Sponsored or accepted: J1 visa

Hawaii

University of Hawaii Obstetrics and Gynecology Residency Program

Specialty: Obstetrics and Gynecology
Program name: University of Hawaii Program
Program code: 220-14-31-081

State: Hawaii
Address: Kapiolani Medical Center for Women and Children

1319 Punahou St, Honolulu, HI 96826
Phone: (808) 203-6518
Fax: (808) 955-2174
Percentage of IMGs in the program: 0% (Occasionally one)
Minimum USMLE Step 1 Score Requirement: No limits set
Minimum USMLE Step 2 Score Requirement: No limits set
Attempts on any step: No limits set
CS required at time of application: Yes including ECFMG certificate
USCE Requirement: Yes 1year
Cut-Off time since graduation: No limits set
Program offers couple match: Yes
Visas Sponsored or accepted: J1 visa

Illinois

Mount Sinai Hospital Medical Center of Chicago Obstetrics and Gynecology Residency Program

Specialty: Obstetrics and Gynecology
Program name: Mount Sinai Hospital Medical Center of Chicago Program
Program code: 220-16-11-088
NRMP Code: 1144220C0
Program type: Community-based university affiliated hospital
State: Illinois
Address: Mount Sinai Hospital Med Center, Department of Ob/Gyn Rm F208,
　　　　　1500 S California Ave, Chicago, IL 60608
Phone: (773) 257-6459
Fax: (773) 257-6359
Percentage of IMGs in the program: 80%
Minimum USMLE Step 1 Score Requirement: No limits set
Minimum USMLE Step 2 Score Requirement: No limits set
Attempts on any step: Must pass on first attempt
CS required at time of application: No
USCE Requirement: None
Cut-Off time since graduation: No limits set
Program offers couple match: Yes
Visas Sponsored or accepted: J1 visa

McGaw Medical Center of Northwestern University Obstetrics and Gynecology Residency Program

Specialty: Obstetrics and Gynecology
Program name: McGaw Medical Center of Northwestern University Program
Program code: 220-16-21-089
NRMP Code: 2247220C0
Program type: University-based
State: Illinois
Address: Prentice Women's Hospital,
        250 E Superior St, Chicago, IL 60611
Phone: (312) 472-4673
Fax: (312) 472-4687
Percentage of IMGs in the program: 5%
Minimum USMLE Step 1 Score Requirement: No limits set
Minimum USMLE Step 2 Score Requirement: No limits set
Attempts on any step: Must pass from first attempt including CS exam
CS required at time of application: No
USCE Requirement: None
Cut-Off time since graduation: No limits set
Program offers couple match: No
Visas Sponsored or accepted: J1 visa and H1b visa

Mercy Hospital and Medical Center Obstetrics and Gynecology Residency Program

Specialty: Obstetrics and Gynecology
Program name: Mercy Hospital and Medical Center Program
Program code: 220-16-11-086
State: Illinois
Address: Mercy Hospital and Medical Center
2525 S Michigan Ave, Chicago, IL 60616-2477
Phone: (312) 567-2490
Fax: (312) 567-2628
Percentage of IMGs in the program: 0%
Minimum USMLE Step 1 Score Requirement: No limits set
Minimum USMLE Step 2 Score Requirement: No limits set
Attempts on any step: Must pass first attempt including CS exam
CS required at time of application: Yes including ECFMG certificate
USCE Requirement: None
Cut-Off time since graduation: 5 years
Program offers couple match: Yes
Visas Sponsored or accepted: No visa

Advocate Illinois Masonic Medical Center Obstetrics and Gynecology Residency Program

Specialty: Obstetrics and Gynecology
Program name: Advocate Illinois Masonic Medical Center Program
Program code: 220-16-21-085
NRMP Code: 1137220C0
Program type: Community-based university affiliated hospital
State: Illinois
Address: Advocate Illinois Masonic Medical Center,
836 W Wellington Ave, Chicago, IL 60657-5193
Phone: (773) 296-5590
Fax: (773) 296-7207
Percentage of IMGs in the program: 0%
Minimum USMLE Step 1 Score Requirement: No limits set
Minimum USMLE Step 2 Score Requirement: No limits set
Attempts on any step: No limits set
CS required at time of application: No
USCE Requirement: None
Cut-Off time since graduation: No limits set
Program offers couple match: Yes
Visas Sponsored or accepted: J1 visa

Rush University Medical Center Obstetrics and Gynecology Residency Program

Specialty: Obstetrics and Gynecology
Program name: Rush University Medical Center Program
Program code: 220-16-21-090
Program type: University-based
State: Illinois
Address: Rush University Medical Center,
1653 W Congress Pkwy, Chicago, IL 60612-3833
Phone: (312) 942-6610
Fax: (312) 942-6606
Percentage of IMGs in the program: 5%
Minimum USMLE Step 1 Score Requirement: 205
Minimum USMLE Step 2 Score Requirement: 205
Attempts on any step: No limits set
CS required at time of application: No
USCE Requirement: None
Cut-Off time since graduation: 2 years
Program offers couple match: Yes
Visas Sponsored or accepted: J1 visa and H1b visa

St. Joseph Hospital Obstetrics and Gynecology Residency Program

Specialty: Obstetrics and Gynecology
Program name: Presence St Joseph Hospital (Chicago) Program
Program code: 220-16-11-091
NRMP Code: 1405220C0
Program type: Community-based university affiliated hospital
State: Illinois
Address: St Joseph Hospital
          2900 N Lake Shore Dr, Chicago, IL 60657
Phone: (773) 665-3132
Fax: (773) 665-3718
Percentage of IMGs in the program: 0%
Minimum USMLE Step 1 Score Requirement: No limits set
Minimum USMLE Step 2 Score Requirement: No limits set
Attempts on any step: Must pass on first attempt
CS required at time of application: Yes including ECFMG certificate
USCE Requirement: None
Cut-Off time since graduation: 3 years
Program offers couple match: No
Visas Sponsored or accepted: J1 visa and H1b visa

University of Chicago Obstetrics and Gynecology Residency Program

Specialty: Obstetrics and Gynecology
Program name: University of Chicago Program
Program code: 220-16-11-092
NRMP Code: 1160220C0
Program type: University-based
State: Illinois
Address: University of Chicago Hospitals,
          5841 S Maryland Ave, Chicago, IL
60637-1470
Phone: (773) 834-0598
Fax: (773) 702-0840
Percentage of IMGs in the program: 0%
Minimum USMLE Step 1 Score Requirement:
No limits set
Minimum USMLE Step 2 Score Requirement:
No limits set
Attempts on any step: Two maximum attempts
on any step.
CS required at time of application: Yes
including ECFMG certificate
USCE Requirement: None
Cut-Off time since graduation: No limits set
Program offers couple match: Yes
Visas Sponsored or accepted: J1 visa and H1b
visa

University of Illinois College of Medicine at Chicago Obstetrics and Gynecology Residency Program

Specialty: Obstetrics and Gynecology
Program name: University of Illinois College of Medicine at Chicago Program
Program code: 220-16-11-093
NRMP Code: 1150220C0
Program type: University-based
State: Illinois
Address: University of Illinois Hospital, 820 S Wood St, Chicago, IL 60612
Phone: (312) 996-0532
Fax: (312) 996-4238
Percentage of IMGs in the program: 0%
Minimum USMLE Step 1 Score Requirement: No limits set
Minimum USMLE Step 2 Score Requirement: No limits set
Attempts on any step: Must pass on first attempt
CS required at time of application: No
USCE Requirement: None
Cut-Off time since graduation: No limits set
Program offers couple match: Yes
Visas Sponsored or accepted: J1 visa

St. Francis Hospital of Evanston Obstetrics and Gynecology Residency Program

Specialty: Obstetrics and Gynecology
Program name: Presence St Francis Hospital Program
Program code: 220-16-21-094
NRMP Code: 1168220C0
Program type: Community-based university affiliated hospital
State: Illinois
Address: St Francis Hospital, Medical Education
355 Ridge Ave, Evanston, IL 60202
Phone: (847) 316-6229
Fax: (847) 316-3307
Percentage of IMGs in the program: 0%
Minimum USMLE Step 1 Score Requirement: No limits set
Minimum USMLE Step 2 Score Requirement: No limits set
Attempts on any step: Maximum of 2 attempts
CS required at time of application: Yes including ECFMG certificate
USCE Requirement: None
Cut-Off time since graduation: No limits set
Program offers couple match: Yes
Visas Sponsored or accepted: J1 visa and H1b visa

Loyola University Obstetrics and Gynecology Residency Program

Specialty: Obstetrics and Gynecology
Program name: Loyola University Program
Program code: 220-16-21-095
NRMP Code: 1170220C0
Program type: University-based
State: Illinois
Address: Loyola University Medical Center,
2160 S First Ave, Maywood, IL 60153
Phone: (708) 216-8078
Fax: (708) 216-2171
Percentage of IMGs in the program: 5%
Minimum USMLE Step 1 Score Requirement:
No limits set
Minimum USMLE Step 2 Score Requirement:
No limits set
Attempts on any step: Two maximum attempts including CS exam.
CS required at time of application: No
USCE Requirement: Yes
Cut-Off time since graduation: 5 years
Program offers couple match: Yes
Visas Sponsored or accepted: J1 visa

Advocate Lutheran General Hospital Obstetrics and Gynecology Residency Program

Specialty: Obstetrics and Gynecology
Program name: Advocate Lutheran General Hospital Program
Program code: 220-16-21-325
NRMP Code: 1176220C0
Program type: Community-based university affiliated hospital
State: Illinois
Address: Advocate Lutheran General Hospital, 1775 W Dempster St, Park Ridge, IL 60068
Phone: (847) 723-8404
Fax: (847) 723-1658
Percentage of IMGs in the program: 0%
Minimum USMLE Step 1 Score Requirement: 205
Minimum USMLE Step 2 Score Requirement: 205
Attempts on any step: Must pass on first attempt including CS exam
CS required at time of application: Yes
USCE Requirement: Yes
Cut-Off time since graduation: 5 years
Program offers couple match: No
Visas Sponsored or accepted: No visa

University of Illinois College of Medicine at Peoria Obstetrics and Gynecology Residency Program

Specialty: Obstetrics and Gynecology
Program name: University of Illinois College of Medicine at Peoria Program
Program code: 220-16-11-096
NRMP Code: 1175220C0
Program type: Community-based university affiliated hospital
State: Illinois
Address: OSF St Francis Medical Center,
530 NE Glen Oak Ave, Peoria, IL 61637
Phone: (309) 655-4163
Fax: (309) 655-3739
Percentage of IMGs in the program: 0%
Minimum USMLE Step 1 Score Requirement: No limits set
Minimum USMLE Step 2 Score Requirement: No limits set
Attempts on any step: No limits set
CS required at time of application: No
USCE Requirement: None
Cut-Off time since graduation: No limits set
Program offers couple match: Yes
Visas Sponsored or accepted: J1 visa and H1b visa

Southern Illinois University Obstetrics and Gynecology Residency Program

Specialty: Obstetrics and Gynecology
Program name: Southern Illinois University Program
Program code: 220-16-21-097
NRMP Code: 2922220C0
Program type: Community-based university affiliated hospital
State: Illinois
Address: Southern Illinois University School of Medicine,

Department of Ob/Gyn PO Box 19640 6W70,

415 N 9th, Springfield, IL 62794-9640
Phone: (217) 545-6498
Fax: (217) 545-7958
Percentage of IMGs in the program: 7%
Minimum USMLE Step 1 Score Requirement: 205
Minimum USMLE Step 2 Score Requirement: 205
Attempts on any step: Must pass on first attempt, might consider 2nd attempt if good score.
CS required at time of application: Yes including ECFMG certificate
USCE Requirement: None
Cut-Off time since graduation: 5 years

Program offers couple match: Yes
Visas Sponsored or accepted: J1 visa

Indiana

St Vincent Hospitals and Health Care Center Obstetrics and Gynecology Residency Program

Specialty: Obstetrics and Gynecology
Program name: St Vincent Hospitals and Health Care Center Program
Program code: 220-17-11-101
State: Indiana
Address: St Vincent Hospital and Health Centers
8111 Township Line Rd, Indianapolis, IN 46260
Phone: (317) 415-7528
Fax: (317) 415-7529
Percentage of IMGs in the program: 0%
Minimum USMLE Step 1 Score Requirement: No limits set
Minimum USMLE Step 2 Score Requirement: No limits set
Attempts on any step: No limits set
CS required at time of application: No
USCE Requirement: Yes

Cut-Off time since graduation: 5 years
Program offers couple match: Yes
Visas Sponsored or accepted: J1 visa

Indiana University School of Medicine Obstetrics and Gynecology Residency Program

Specialty: Obstetrics and Gynecology
Program name: Indiana University School of Medicine Program
Program code: 220-17-21-099
NRMP Code: 1187220C0
Program type: University-based
State: Indiana
Address: Indiana University Medical Center
550 N University Blvd, Indianapolis, IN 46202
Phone: (317) 948-5923
Fax: (317) 948-7454
Percentage of IMGs in the program: 0%
Minimum USMLE Step 1 Score Requirement: No limits set
Minimum USMLE Step 2 Score Requirement: No limits set
Attempts on any step: No limits set
CS required at time of application: Yes including ECFMG certificate
USCE Requirement: Yes
Cut-Off time since graduation: 3 years

Program offers couple match: Yes
Visas Sponsored or accepted: J1 visa

Iowa

University of Iowa Hospitals and Clinics Obstetrics and Gynecology Residency Program

Specialty: Obstetrics and Gynecology
Program name: University of Iowa Hospitals and Clinics Program
Program code: 220-18-21-102
NRMP Code: 1203220C0
Program type: University-based
State: Iowa
Address: University of Iowa Hospitals and Clinics
      200 Hawkins Dr, Iowa City, IA 52242
Phone: (319) 356-4403
Fax: (319) 384-8620
Percentage of IMGs in the program: 0%
Minimum USMLE Step 1 Score Requirement: No limits set
Minimum USMLE Step 2 Score Requirement: No limits set

Attempts on any step: Must pass on first attempt including CS exam
CS required at time of application: No
USCE Requirement: None
Cut-Off time since graduation: No limits set
Program offers couple match: Yes
Visas Sponsored or accepted: J1 visa and H1b visa

Kansas

University of Kansas School of Medicine Obstetrics and Gynecology Residency Program

Specialty: Obstetrics and Gynecology
Program name: University of Kansas School of Medicine Program
Program code: 220-19-11-103
NRMP Code: 1208220C0
Program type: University-based
State: Kansas
Address: University of Kansas Medical Center
        3901 Rainbow Blvd, Kansas City, KS 66160-7316
Phone: (913) 588-6245

Fax: (913) 588-6271
Percentage of IMGs in the program: 0%
Minimum USMLE Step 1 Score Requirement: No limits set
Minimum USMLE Step 2 Score Requirement: No limits set
Attempts on any step: No limits set
CS required at time of application: Yes
USCE Requirement: None
Cut-Off time since graduation: 5 years
Program offers couple match: Yes
Visas Sponsored or accepted: J1 visa

University of Kansas (Wichita) Obstetrics and Gynecology Residency Program

Specialty: Obstetrics and Gynecology
Program name: University of Kansas (Wichita) Program
Program code: 220-19-11-104
State: Kansas
Address: Wesley Medical Center
550 N Hillside, Wichita, KS 67214
Phone: (316) 962-3182
Fax: (316) 962-7396
Percentage of IMGs in the program: 0%
Minimum USMLE Step 1 Score Requirement: No limits set

Minimum USMLE Step 2 Score Requirement: No limits set
Attempts on any step: No limits set
CS required at time of application: Yes including ECFMG certificate
USCE Requirement: None
Cut-Off time since graduation: 5 years
Program offers couple match: Yes
Visas Sponsored or accepted: J1 visa

Kentucky

University of Louisville Obstetrics and Gynecology Residency Program

Specialty: Obstetrics and Gynecology
Program name: University of Louisville Program
Program code: 220-20-21-106
NRMP Code: 1217220C0
Program type: University-based
State: Kentucky
Address: University of Louisville Hospital
550 S Jackson St, Louisville, KY 40202

Phone: (502) 561-7448
Fax: (502) 561-7480
Percentage of IMGs in the program: 0%
Minimum USMLE Step 1 Score Requirement: 215
Minimum USMLE Step 2 Score Requirement: 215
Attempts on any step: No limits set
CS required at time of application: No
USCE Requirement: None
Cut-Off time since graduation: No limits set
Program offers couple match: Yes
Visas Sponsored or accepted: J1 visa

University of Kentucky College of Medicine Obstetrics and Gynecology Residency Program

Specialty: Obstetrics and Gynecology
Program name: University of Kentucky College of Medicine Program
Program code: 220-20-11-105
State: Kentucky
Address: University of Kentucky Medical Center
800 Rose St, Lexington, KY 40536-0293
Phone: (859) 218-1661
Fax: (859) 257-3181
Percentage of IMGs in the program: 0%
Minimum USMLE Step 1 Score Requirement: No limits set

Minimum USMLE Step 2 Score Requirement:
No limits set
Attempts on any step: Must pass on maximum
the 3rd attempt
CS required at time of application: No
USCE Requirement: None
Cut-Off time since graduation: No limits set
Program offers couple match: Yes
Visas Sponsored or accepted: No visa

Louisiana

Louisiana State University (Shreveport) Obstetrics and Gynecology Residency Program

Specialty: Obstetrics and Gynecology
Program name: Louisiana State University
(Shreveport) Program
Program code: 220-21-11-110
NRMP Code: 1232220C0
Program type: University-based
State: Louisiana
Address: LSU Health Sciences Center
Shreveport
        1501 Kings Hwy, Shreveport, LA
71130-3932

Phone: (318) 675-8295
Fax: (318) 675-4671
Percentage of IMGs in the program: 25%
Minimum USMLE Step 1 Score Requirement: No limits set
Minimum USMLE Step 2 Score Requirement: No limits set
Attempts on any step: Must pass on first attempt including CS exam
CS required at time of application: Yes including ECFMG certificate
USCE Requirement: Yes
Cut-Off time since graduation: 5 years
Program offers couple match: Yes
Visas Sponsored or accepted: J1 visa

Louisiana State University (Baton Rouge)Obstetrics and Gynecology Residency Program

Specialty: Obstetrics and Gynecology
Program name: Louisiana State University (Baton Rouge) Program
Program code: 220-21-13-364
NRMP Code: 1221220C0
Program type: University-based
State: Louisiana
Address: Louisiana State University
        500 Rue de la Vie, Baton Rouge, LA 70817

Phone: (225) 215-7442
Fax: (225) 922-3382
Percentage of IMGs in the program: 20%
Minimum USMLE Step 1 Score Requirement: No limits set
Minimum USMLE Step 2 Score Requirement: No limits set
Attempts on any step: No limits set
CS required at time of application: Yes including ECFMG certificate
USCE Requirement: None
Cut-Off time since graduation: No limits set
Program offers couple match: Yes
Visas Sponsored or accepted: J1 visa

Louisiana State University Obstetrics and Gynecology Residency Program

Specialty: Obstetrics and Gynecology
Program name: Louisiana State University Program
Program code: 220-21-21-107
NRMP Code: 1224220C0
Program type: University-based
State: Louisiana
Address: LSU Health Science Center New Orleans
      1542 Tulane Ave, New Orleans, LA 70112

Phone: (504) 568-4890
Fax: (504) 568-6496
Percentage of IMGs in the program: 10%
Minimum USMLE Step 1 Score Requirement: 220
Minimum USMLE Step 2 Score Requirement: 220
Attempts on any step: No limits set
CS required at time of application: Yes including ECFMG certificate
USCE Requirement: Yes 1 month
Cut-Off time since graduation: No limits set
Program offers couple match: Yes
Visas Sponsored or accepted: J1 visa

Tulane University Obstetrics and Gynecology Residency Program

Specialty: Obstetrics and Gynecology
Program name: Tulane University Program
Program code: 220-21-21-108
NRMP Code: 3073220C0
Program type: University-based
State: Louisiana
Address: Tulane University Health Sciences Center

    1430 Tulane Ave, New Orleans, LA 70118-2699
Phone: (504) 988-5216

Fax: (504) 988-1846
Percentage of IMGs in the program: 0%
Minimum USMLE Step 1 Score Requirement:
No limits set
Minimum USMLE Step 2 Score Requirement:
No limits set
Attempts on any step: Must pass on first
attempt
CS required at time of application: Yes
including ECFMG certificate
USCE Requirement: Yes
Cut-Off time since graduation: 3 years
Program offers couple match: Yes
Visas Sponsored or accepted: No visa

Ochsner Clinic Foundation Obstetrics and Gynecology Residency Program

Specialty: Obstetrics and Gynecology
Program name: Ochsner Clinic Foundation
Program
Program code: 220-21-22-109
NRMP Code: 1966220C0
Program type: Community-based
State: Louisiana
Address: Ochsner Clinic Foundation
          2700 Napoleon Ave, New Orleans, LA
70115
Phone: (504) 842-3173

Fax: (504) 842-4152
Percentage of IMGs in the program: 10%
Minimum USMLE Step 1 Score Requirement:
No limits set
Minimum USMLE Step 2 Score Requirement:
No limits set
Attempts on any step: No limits set
CS required at time of application: Yes
including ECFMG certificate
USCE Requirement: None
Cut-Off time since graduation: 5 years
Program offers couple match: Yes
Visas Sponsored or accepted: No visa

Maine

Maine Medical Center Obstetrics and Gynecology Residency Program

Specialty: Obstetrics and Gynecology
Program name: Maine Medical Center Program
Program code: 220-22-11-111
NRMP Code: 1236220C0
Program type: Community-based university affiliated hospital
State: Maine

Address: Maine Medical Center
          22 Bramhall St, Portland, ME 04102
Phone: (207) 662-2749
Fax: (207) 662-6252
Percentage of IMGs in the program: 0%
Minimum USMLE Step 1 Score Requirement:
No limits set
Minimum USMLE Step 2 Score Requirement:
No limits set
Attempts on any step: No limits set
CS required at time of application: No
USCE Requirement: None
Cut-Off time since graduation: No limits set
Program offers couple match: Yes
Visas Sponsored or accepted: J1 visa

Maryland

University of Maryland Obstetrics and Gynecology Residency Program

Specialty: Obstetrics and Gynecology
Program name: University of Maryland Program
Program code: 220-23-21-121

NRMP Code: 1252220C0
Program type: University-based
State: Maryland
Address: University of Maryland Medical System
            22 S Greene St, Baltimore, MD 21201
Phone: (410) 328-5959
Fax: (410) 328-0279
Percentage of IMGs in the program: 0%
Minimum USMLE Step 1 Score Requirement: 200
Minimum USMLE Step 2 Score Requirement: 210
Attempts on any step: Must pass on first attempt including CS exam
CS required at time of application: Yes including ECFMG certificate
USCE Requirement: None
Cut-Off time since graduation: 5 years
Program offers couple match: Yes
Visas Sponsored or accepted: J1 visa

Johns Hopkins University Obstetrics and Gynecology Residency Program

Specialty: Obstetrics and Gynecology
Program name: Johns Hopkins University Program
Program code: 220-23-21-114

NRMP Code: 1242220C0
Program type: University-based
State: Maryland
Address: Johns Hopkins Hospital
              600 N Wolfe St, Baltimore, MD 21287
Phone: (410) 955-6710
Fax: (410) 502-6683
Percentage of IMGs in the program: 0%
Minimum USMLE Step 1 Score Requirement:
No limits set
Minimum USMLE Step 2 Score Requirement:
No limits set
Attempts on any step: No limits set
CS required at time of application: Yes
including ECFMG certificate
USCE Requirement: None
Cut-Off time since graduation: No limits set
Program offers couple match: Yes
Visas Sponsored or accepted: J1 visa

MedStar Franklin Square Hospital Center Obstetrics and Gynecology Residency Program

Specialty: Obstetrics and Gynecology
Program name: MedStar Franklin Square
Hospital Center Program
Program code: 220-23-21-112

NRMP Code: 1240220C0
Program type: Community-based
State: Maryland
Address: MedStar Franklin Square Medical
Center
          9000 Franklin Square Dr, Baltimore,
MD 21237-3998
Phone: (443) 777-7062
Fax: (443) 777-8180
Percentage of IMGs in the program: 60%
Minimum USMLE Step 1 Score Requirement:
No limits set
Minimum USMLE Step 2 Score Requirement:
No limits set
Attempts on any step: No limits set
CS required at time of application: No
USCE Requirement: None
Cut-Off time since graduation: No limits set
Program offers couple match: Yes
Visas Sponsored or accepted: J1 visa

Sinai Hospital of Baltimore Obstetrics and Gynecology Residency Program

Specialty: Obstetrics and Gynecology
Program name: Sinai Hospital of Baltimore
Program
Program code: 220-23-12-118

NRMP Code: 1249220C0
Program type: Community-based
State: Maryland
Address: Sinai Hospital of Baltimore
2401 W Belvedere Ave, Baltimore, MD 21215-5271
Phone: (410) 601-9197
Fax: (410) 601-8862
Percentage of IMGs in the program: 0%
Minimum USMLE Step 1 Score Requirement: 210
Minimum USMLE Step 2 Score Requirement: 210
Attempts on any step: Must pass on first attempt including CS exam
CS required at time of application: Yes including ECFMG certificate
USCE Requirement: None
Cut-Off time since graduation: 5 years
Program offers couple match: Yes
Visas Sponsored or accepted: J1 visa

Massachusetts

Beth Israel Deaconess Medical Center Obstetrics and Gynecology Residency Program

Specialty: Obstetrics and Gynecology
Program name: Beth Israel Deaconess Medical Center Program
Program code: 220-24-11-123
NRMP Code: 1256220C0
Program type: University-based
State: Massachusetts
Address: Beth Israel Deaconess Medical Center, 330 Brookline Ave, Boston, MA 02215
Phone: (617) 667-2285
Fax: (617) 667-0842
Percentage of IMGs in the program: 0%
Minimum USMLE Step 1 Score Requirement: 220
Minimum USMLE Step 2 Score Requirement: 220
Attempts on any step: No limits set
CS required at time of application: Yes including ECFMG certificate
USCE Requirement: Yes 1 year
Cut-Off time since graduation: 3 years
Program offers couple match: Yes
Visas Sponsored or accepted: J1 visa

Brigham and Women's Hospital/Massachusetts General Hospital Obstetrics and Gynecology Residency Program

Specialty: Obstetrics and Gynecology
Program name: Brigham and Women's Hospital/Massachusetts General Hospital Program
Program code: 220-24-11-125
NRMP Code: 1265220C0
Program type: University-based
State: Massachusetts
Address: Brigham and Women's Hospital,
          75 Francis St, Boston, MA 02115
Phone: (617) 732-7801
Fax: (617) 730-2833
Percentage of IMGs in the program: 0%
Minimum USMLE Step 1 Score Requirement: No limits set
Minimum USMLE Step 2 Score Requirement: No limits set
Attempts on any step: Must pass maximum on 2nd attempt
CS required at time of application: Yes including ECFMG certificate
USCE Requirement: None
Cut-Off time since graduation: No limits set
Program offers couple match: Yes
Visas Sponsored or accepted: H1b visa

Baystate Medical Center/Tufts University School of Medicine Obstetrics and Gynecology Residency Program

Specialty: Obstetrics and Gynecology
Program name: Baystate Medical Center/Tufts University School of Medicine Program
Program code: 220-24-12-129
NRMP Code: 1286220C0
Program type: Community-based university affiliated hospital
State: Massachusetts
Address: Baystate Medical Center, Department of Ob/Gyn,

759 Chestnut St, Springfield, MA 01199
Phone: (413) 794-5321
Fax: (413) 794-8166
Percentage of IMGs in the program: 20%
Minimum USMLE Step 1 Score Requirement: 220
Minimum USMLE Step 2 Score Requirement: 220
Attempts on any step: Must pass on first attempt
CS required at time of application: No
USCE Requirement: Yes 1 year
Cut-Off time since graduation: No limits set
Program offers couple match: Yes

Visas Sponsored or accepted: J1 visa

Boston Medical Center Obstetrics and Gynecology Residency Program

Specialty: Obstetrics and Gynecology
Program name: Boston Medical Center Program
Program code: 220-24-21-124
NRMP Code: 1257220C0
Program type: University-based
State: Massachusetts
Address: Boston University Medical Center,
          85 E Concord St, Boston, MA 02118
Phone: (617) 414-5166
Fax: (617) 414-7300
Percentage of IMGs in the program: 0%
Minimum USMLE Step 1 Score Requirement:
No limits set
Minimum USMLE Step 2 Score Requirement:
No limits set
Attempts on any step: No limits set
CS required at time of application: Yes
including ECFMG certificate
USCE Requirement: None
Cut-Off time since graduation: No limits set
Program offers couple match: Yes
Visas Sponsored or accepted: J1 visa

Tufts Medical Center Obstetrics and Gynecology Residency Program

Specialty: Obstetrics and Gynecology
Program name: Tufts Medical Center Program
Program code: 220-24-21-128
NRMP Code: 1263220C0
Program type: University-based
State: Massachusetts
Address: Tufts Medical Center,
            800 Washington St, Boston, MA 02111
Phone: (617) 636-0265
Fax: (617) 636-8315
Percentage of IMGs in the program: 20%
Minimum USMLE Step 1 Score Requirement: No limits set
Minimum USMLE Step 2 Score Requirement: No limits set
Attempts on any step: No limits set
CS required at time of application: Yes including ECFMG certificate
USCE Requirement: None
Cut-Off time since graduation: 6 years
Program offers couple match: Yes
Visas Sponsored or accepted: J1 visa

University of Massachusetts
Obstetrics and Gynecology
Residency Program

Specialty: Obstetrics and Gynecology
Program name: University of Massachusetts Program
Program code: 220-24-21-130
NRMP Code: 3050220C0
Program type: University-based
State: Massachusetts
Address: UMass Memorial Medical Center, Department of Ob/Gyn,
           119 Belmont St, Worcester, MA 01605
Phone: (508) 334-8459
Fax: (508) 334-5371
Percentage of IMGs in the program: 10%
Minimum USMLE Step 1 Score Requirement: No limits set
Minimum USMLE Step 2 Score Requirement: No limits set
Attempts on any step: Must pass maximum on 2nd attempt
CS required at time of application: Yes including ECFMG certificate
USCE Requirement: Yes, 1 year
Cut-Off time since graduation: No limits set
Program offers couple match: Yes
Visas Sponsored or accepted: J1 visa

Michigan

Henry Ford Hospital/Wayne State University Obstetrics and Gynecology Residency Program

Specialty: Obstetrics and Gynecology
Program name: Henry Ford Hospital/Wayne State University Program
Program code: 220-25-11-136
NRMP Code: 1300220C0
Program type: Community-based university affiliated hospital
State: Michigan
Address: Henry Ford Hospital
3031 W Grand Blvd, Detroit, MI 48202
Phone: (313) 916-1023
Fax: (313) 916-5008
Percentage of IMGs in the program: 90%
Minimum USMLE Step 1 Score Requirement: 210
Minimum USMLE Step 2 Score Requirement: 210
Attempts on any step: Must pass on the first attempt
CS required at time of application: No but should be scheduled already at time of interview

USCE Requirement: None
Cut-Off time since graduation: 5 years
Program offers couple match: Yes
Visas Sponsored or accepted: J1 visa

St John Hospital and Medical Center Obstetrics and Gynecology Residency Program

Specialty: Obstetrics and Gynecology
Program name: St John Hospital and Medical Center Program
Program code: 220-25-11-137
NRMP Code: 1915220C0
Program type: Community-based university affiliated hospital
State: Michigan
Address: St John Hospital and Medical Center
          19251 Mack Ave, Grosse Pointe Woods, MI 48236
Phone: (313) 343-7798
Fax: (313) 343-7840
Percentage of IMGs in the program: 50%
Minimum USMLE Step 1 Score Requirement: No limits set
Minimum USMLE Step 2 Score Requirement: No limits set

Attempts on any step: Must pass on the first attempt
CS required at time of application: No
USCE Requirement: 1 year
Cut-Off time since graduation: 5 years
Program offers couple match: Yes
Visas Sponsored or accepted: J1 visa

William Beaumont Hospital Obstetrics and Gynecology Residency Program

Specialty: Obstetrics and Gynecology
Program name: William Beaumont Hospital Program
Program code: 220-25-11-146
State: Michigan
Address: Beaumont Health System
3535 W 13 Mile Rd, Royal Oak, MI 48073
Phone: (248) 551-0845
Fax: (248) 551-5010
Percentage of IMGs in the program: 15%
Minimum USMLE Step 1 Score Requirement: No limits set
Minimum USMLE Step 2 Score Requirement: No limits set
Attempts on any step: No limits set
CS required at time of application: No
USCE Requirement: None

Cut-Off time since graduation: No limits set
Program offers couple match: Yes
Visas Sponsored or accepted: J1 visa

Grand Rapids Medical Education Partners/Michigan State University Obstetrics and Gynecology Residency Program

Specialty: Obstetrics and Gynecology
Program name: Grand Rapids Medical Education Partners/Michigan State University Program
Program code: 220-25-21-141
NRMP Code: 2077220C0
Program type: Community-based university affiliated hospital
State: Michigan
Address: Grand Rapids Med Education Partners
330 Barclay NE, Grand Rapids, MI 49503
Phone: (616) 391-1929
Fax: (616) 391-3174
Percentage of IMGs in the program: 40%
Minimum USMLE Step 1 Score Requirement: 210
Minimum USMLE Step 2 Score Requirement: 210

Attempts on any step: Must pass on the first attempt
CS required at time of application: No
USCE Requirement: None
Cut-Off time since graduation: 3 years
Program offers couple match: Yes
Visas Sponsored or accepted: J1 visa

Central Michigan University College of Medicine Obstetrics and Gynecology Residency Program

Specialty: Obstetrics and Gynecology
Program name: Central Michigan University College of Medicine Program
Program code: 220-25-21-147
NRMP Code: 1320220C0
Program type: University-based
State: Michigan
Address: Central Michigan University College of Medicine
          1000 Houghton Ave, Saginaw, MI 48602
Phone: (989) 583-6828
Fax: (989) 583-6941
Percentage of IMGs in the program: 20%
Minimum USMLE Step 1 Score Requirement: 210

**Minimum USMLE Step 2 Score
Requirement:** 210
Attempts on any step: Must pass on the
first attempt
CS required at time of application: Yes
including ECFMG certificate
USCE Requirement: None
Cut-Off time since graduation: 2 years
Program offers couple match: Yes
Visas Sponsored or accepted: J1 visa

Providence Hospital and Medical Centers Obstetrics and Gynecology Residency Program

Specialty: Obstetrics and Gynecology
Program name: Providence Hospital and
Medical Centers Program
Program code: 220-25-21-148
NRMP Code: 1303220C0
Program type: Community-based university
affiliated hospital
State: Michigan
Address: Providence Hospital and Medical
Center
        16001 W Nine Mile Rd, Southfield, MI
48075-4818
Phone: (248) 849-3014
Fax: (248) 849-5398
Percentage of IMGs in the program: 50%

Minimum USMLE Step 1 Score Requirement: 210
Minimum USMLE Step 2 Score Requirement: 210
Attempts on any step: Must pass on the first attempt
CS required at time of application: Yes including ECFMG certificate
USCE Requirement: 1 year
Cut-Off time since graduation: 5 years
Program offers couple match: Yes
Visas Sponsored or accepted: J1 visa

St Joseph Mercy Hospital Obstetrics and Gynecology Residency Program

Specialty: Obstetrics and Gynecology
Program name: St Joseph Mercy Hospital Program
Program code: 220-25-31-131
NRMP Code: 1292220C0
Program type: Community-based university affiliated hospital
State: Michigan
Address: St Joseph Mercy Hospital
            5333 McAuley Dr, Ypsilanti, MI 48197
Phone: (734) 712-5171
Fax: (734) 712-4151
Percentage of IMGs in the program: 20%

Minimum USMLE Step 1 Score Requirement: 210
Minimum USMLE Step 2 Score Requirement: 210
Attempts on any step: No limits set
CS required at time of application: Yes including ECFMG certificate
USCE Requirement: 1-2 months
Cut-Off time since graduation: 2 years
Program offers couple match: Yes
Visas Sponsored or accepted: J1 visa

University of Michigan Obstetrics and Gynecology Residency Program

Specialty: Obstetrics and Gynecology
Program name: University of Michigan Program
Program code: 220-25-31-132
NRMP Code: 1293220C0
Program type: University-based
State: Michigan
Address: University of Michigan Health Systems
          1500 E Medical Center Dr, Ann Arbor, MI 48109-5276
Phone: (734) 936-9434
Fax: (734) 232-6020
Percentage of IMGs in the program: 0%

Minimum USMLE Step 1 Score Requirement: 210
Minimum USMLE Step 2 Score Requirement: 210
Attempts on any step: Must pass on the first attempt
CS required at time of application: Yes including ECFMG certificate
USCE Requirement: None
Cut-Off time since graduation: No limits set
Program offers couple match: Yes
Visas Sponsored or accepted: J1 visa

Oakwood Hospital Obstetrics and Gynecology Residency Program

Specialty: Obstetrics and Gynecology
Program name: Oakwood Hospital Program
Program code: 220-25-31-133
NRMP Code: 1946220C0
Program type: Community-based university affiliated hospital
State: Michigan
Address: Oakwood Hospital and Medical Center
          18101 Oakwood Blvd, Dearborn, MI
48124
Phone: (313) 436-2582
Fax: (313) 436-2783
Percentage of IMGs in the program: 50%

Minimum USMLE Step 1 Score Requirement: 210
Minimum USMLE Step 2 Score Requirement: 210
Attempts on any step: Must pass maximum from the 2nd attempt
CS required at time of application: Yes including ECFMG certificate
USCE Requirement: 1 year
Cut-Off time since graduation: 5 years
Program offers couple match: Yes
Visas Sponsored or accepted: No visa

Hurley Medical Center/Michigan State University Obstetrics and Gynecology Residency Program

Specialty: Obstetrics and Gynecology
Program name: Hurley Medical Center/Michigan State University Program
Program code: 220-25-31-140
NRMP Code: 1307220C0
Program type: Community-based university affiliated hospital
State: Michigan
Address: Hurley Medical Center
            One Hurley Plaza, Flint, MI 48503-5993
Phone: (810) 262-6426
Fax: (810) 257-9076

Percentage of IMGs in the program: 80%
Minimum USMLE Step 1 Score Requirement: 215
Minimum USMLE Step 2 Score Requirement: 220
Attempts on any step: Must pass maximum from the 2nd attempt
CS required at time of application: Yes including ECFMG certificate
USCE Requirement: None
Cut-Off time since graduation: 7 years
Program offers couple match: Yes
Visas Sponsored or accepted: J1 visa

Sparrow Hospital/Michigan State University Obstetrics and Gynecology Residency Program

Specialty: Obstetrics and Gynecology
Program name: Sparrow Hospital/Michigan State University Program
Program code: 220-25-31-143
NRMP Code: 1315220C0
Program type: Community-based university affiliated hospital
State: Michigan
Address: Sparrow Hospital
        1215 E Michigan Ave, Lansing, MI 48909-7980
Phone: (517) 364-2577

Fax: (517) 364-2222
Percentage of IMGs in the program: 40%
Minimum USMLE Step 1 Score Requirement: 210
Minimum USMLE Step 2 Score Requirement: 210
Attempts on any step: No limits set
CS required at time of application: Yes including ECFMG certificate
USCE Requirement: None unless you graduated more than 2 years ago
Cut-Off time since graduation: None but must be clinically active within the last 2 years
Program offers couple match: Yes
Visas Sponsored or accepted: J1 visa

Detroit Medical Center/Wayne State University Obstetrics and Gynecology Residency Program

Specialty: Obstetrics and Gynecology
Program name: Detroit Medical Center/Wayne State University Program
Program code: 220-25-31-358
NRMP Code: 1295220C0
Program type: University-based
State: Michigan
Address: Hutzel Women's Hospital
          3990 John R St, Detroit, MI 48021
Phone: (313) 993-4030

Fax: (313) 993-4116
Percentage of IMGs in the program: 30%
Minimum USMLE Step 1 Score Requirement:
No limits set
Minimum USMLE Step 2 Score Requirement:
No limits set
Attempts on any step: Must pass on the first attempt
CS required at time of application: Yes including ECFMG certificate
USCE Requirement: None
Cut-Off time since graduation: 5 years
Program offers couple match: Yes
Visas Sponsored or accepted: J1 visa

Minnesota

University of Minnesota Obstetrics and Gynecology Residency Program

Specialty: Obstetrics and Gynecology
Program name: University of Minnesota Program
Program code: 220-26-21-149
NRMP Code: 1334220C0
Program type: University-based
State: Minnesota

Address: University of Minnesota Medical School

　　　　420 Delaware St SE, Minneapolis, MN 55455

Phone: (612) 301-3417
Fax: (612) 301-3416
Percentage of IMGs in the program: 0%
Minimum USMLE Step 1 Score Requirement: No limits set
Minimum USMLE Step 2 Score Requirement: No limits set
Attempts on any step: Must pass on the first attempt
CS required at time of application: Yes including ECFMG certificate
USCE Requirement: 6 months
Cut-Off time since graduation: 5 years unless clinically active
Program offers couple match: Yes
Visas Sponsored or accepted: J1 visa

Mayo Clinic College of Medicine (Rochester) Obstetrics and Gynecology Residency Program

Specialty: Obstetrics and Gynecology
Program name: Mayo Clinic College of Medicine (Rochester) Program
Program code: 220-26-21-150
NRMP Code: 1328220C1, 1328220C0

Program type: University-based
State: Minnesota
Address: Mayo Clinic
            200 First St SW, Rochester, MN 55905
Phone: (507) 266-3262
Fax: (507) 266-7953
Percentage of IMGs in the program: 20%
Minimum USMLE Step 1 Score Requirement: 215
Minimum USMLE Step 2 Score Requirement: 215
Attempts on any step: Must pass on the first attempt
CS required at time of application: Yes including ECFMG certificate
USCE Requirement: 2 months
Cut-Off time since graduation: 10 years
Program offers couple match: Yes
Visas Sponsored or accepted: J1 visa and H1b visa

Mississippi

University of Mississippi Medical Center Obstetrics and Gynecology Residency Program

Specialty: Obstetrics and Gynecology
Program name: University of Mississippi Medical Center Program
Program code: 220-27-11-151
NRMP Code: 1957220C0
Program type: University-based
State: Mississippi
Address: University of Mississippi Medical Center
            2500 N State St, Jackson, MS 39216
Phone: (601) 984-5339
Fax: (601) 984-4566
Percentage of IMGs in the program: 10%
Minimum USMLE Step 1 Score Requirement: 220
Minimum USMLE Step 2 Score Requirement: 220
Attempts on any step: No limits set
CS required at time of application: No
USCE Requirement: None
Cut-Off time since graduation: No limits set
Program offers couple match: Yes
Visas Sponsored or accepted: J1 visa

Missouri

University of Missouri-Columbia Obstetrics and Gynecology Residency Program

Specialty: Obstetrics and Gynecology
Program name: University of Missouri-Columbia Program
Program code: 220-28-11-152
NRMP Code: 1994220C0
Program type: University-based
State: Missouri
Address: University of Missouri-Columbia
500 N Keene St, Columbia, MO 65201
Phone: (573) 817-3096
Fax: (573) 817-6645
Percentage of IMGs in the program: 0%
Minimum USMLE Step 1 Score Requirement: 210
Minimum USMLE Step 2 Score Requirement: 210
Attempts on any step: No limits set
CS required at time of application: No
USCE Requirement: None
Cut-Off time since graduation: No limits set
Program offers couple match: Yes
Visas Sponsored or accepted: No visa

University of Missouri at Kansas City Obstetrics and Gynecology Residency Program

Specialty: Obstetrics and Gynecology
Program name: University of Missouri at Kansas City Program
Program code: 220-28-21-154
NRMP Code: 1343220C0,
Program type: Community-based university affiliated hospital
State: Missouri
Address: Truman Medical Center
            2301 Holmes St, Kansas City, MO 64108
Phone: (816) 404-0886
Fax: (816) 404-0888
Percentage of IMGs in the program: 10%
Minimum USMLE Step 1 Score Requirement: No limits set
Minimum USMLE Step 2 Score Requirement: No limits set
Attempts on any step: No limits set
CS required at time of application: Yes including ECFMG certificate
USCE Requirement: None
Cut-Off time since graduation: 3 years
Program offers couple match: Yes
Visas Sponsored or accepted: J1 visa

Washington University/B-JH/SLCH Consortium Obstetrics and Gynecology Residency Program

Specialty: Obstetrics and Gynecology
Program name: Washington University/B-JH/SLCH Consortium Program
Program code: 220-28-21-155
State: Missouri
Address: Washington University School of Medicine

4911 Barnes-Jewish Hospital Plaza, St Louis, MO 63110
Phone: (314) 362-1016
Fax: (314) 747-1490
Percentage of IMGs in the program: 0%
Minimum USMLE Step 1 Score Requirement: No limits set
Minimum USMLE Step 2 Score Requirement: No limits set
Attempts on any step: No limits set
CS required at time of application: Yes including ECFMG certificate
USCE Requirement: None
Cut-Off time since graduation: No limits set
Program offers couple match: Yes
Visas Sponsored or accepted: J1 visa

Mercy Hospital (St Louis) Obstetrics and Gynecology Residency Program

Specialty: Obstetrics and Gynecology
Program name: Mercy Hospital (St Louis) Program
Program code: 220-28-22-157
NRMP Code: 1362220C0
Program type: Community-based
State: Missouri
Address: Mercy Hospital St Louis
          615 S New Ballas Rd, St Louis, MO 63141
Phone: (314) 251-6826
Fax: (314) 251-4376
Percentage of IMGs in the program: 5%
Minimum USMLE Step 1 Score Requirement: 220
Minimum USMLE Step 2 Score Requirement: 220
Attempts on any step: Must pass on the first attempt
CS required at time of application: No
USCE Requirement: None
Cut-Off time since graduation: 5 years
Program offers couple match: Yes
Visas Sponsored or accepted: H1b visa

St Louis University School of Medicine Obstetrics and Gynecology Residency Program

Specialty: Obstetrics and Gynecology
Program name: St Louis University School of Medicine Program
Program code: 220-28-22-158
NRMP Code: 1365220C0
Program type: University-based
State: Missouri
Address: St Mary's Health Center
6420 Clayton Rd, St Louis, MO 63117
Phone: (314) 781-4772 Ext: 7
Fax: (314) 645-8771
Percentage of IMGs in the program: 0%
Minimum USMLE Step 1 Score Requirement: No limits set
Minimum USMLE Step 2 Score Requirement: No limits set
Attempts on any step: No limits set
CS required at time of application: Yes including ECFMG certificate
USCE Requirement: None
Cut-Off time since graduation: No limits set
Program offers couple match: Yes
Visas Sponsored or accepted: J1 visa

Nebraska

Creighton University Obstetrics and Gynecology Residency Program

Specialty: Obstetrics and Gynecology OB GYN Residency
Program name: Creighton University Program
Program code: 220-30-21-160
NRMP Code: 1372220C0
Program type: University-based
State: Nebraska
Address: Alegent Creighton University Medical Center
    601 N 30th St, Omaha, NE 68131
Phone: (402) 280-4438
Fax: (402) 280-4315
Percentage of IMGs in the program: 5%
Minimum USMLE Step 1 Score Requirement: No limits set
Minimum USMLE Step 2 Score Requirement: No limits set
Attempts on any step: No limits set
CS required at time of application: No
USCE Requirement: None
Cut-Off time since graduation: No limits set
Program offers couple match: Yes
Visas Sponsored or accepted: No visa

University of Nebraska Medical Center College of Medicine Obstetrics and Gynecology Residency Program

Specialty: Obstetrics and Gynecology OB GYN Residency
Program name: University of Nebraska Medical Center College of Medicine Program
Program code: 220-30-21-161
NRMP Code: 1376220C0
Program type: University-based
State: Nebraska
Address: University of Nebraska Medical Center
983255 Nebraska Medical Center, Omaha, NE 68198-3255
Phone: (402) 559-6160
Fax: (402) 559-9080
Percentage of IMGs in the program: 0%
Minimum USMLE Step 1 Score Requirement: No limits set
Minimum USMLE Step 2 Score Requirement: No limits set
Attempts on any step: No limits set
CS required at time of application: Yes including ECFMG certificate
USCE Requirement: None
Cut-Off time since graduation: 5 years

Program offers couple match: Yes
Visas Sponsored or accepted: J1 visa

Nevada

University of Nevada School of Medicine (Las Vegas) Obstetrics and Gynecology Residency Program

Specialty: Obstetrics and Gynecology OB GYN Residency
Program name: University of Nevada School of Medicine (Las Vegas) Program
Program code: 220-31-21-318
NRMP Code: 2028220C0
Program type: Community-based university affiliated hospital
State: Nevada
Address: University of Nevada School of Medicine
          2040 W Charleston Blvd, Las Vegas, NV 89102
Phone: (702) 671-2385
Fax: (702) 671-2333
Percentage of IMGs in the program: 20%

Minimum USMLE Step 1 Score Requirement:
No limits set
Minimum USMLE Step 2 Score Requirement:
No limits set
Attempts on any step: No limits set
CS required at time of application: Yes
including ECFMG certificate
USCE Requirement: None
Cut-Off time since graduation: 5 years
Program offers couple match: Yes
Visas Sponsored or accepted: J1 visa

New Hampshire

Dartmouth-Hitchcock Medical Center Obstetrics and Gynecology Residency Program

Specialty: Obstetrics and Gynecology OB GYN
Residency
Program name: Dartmouth-Hitchcock Medical
Center Program
Program code: 220-32-12-352
NRMP Code: 1377220C0
Program type: University-based
State: New Hampshire

Address: Dartmouth-Hitchcock Medical Center
One Medical Center Dr, Lebanon, NH 03756
Phone: (603) 653-9289
Fax: (603) 650-0906
Percentage of IMGs in the program: 0% (occasionally 1 match)
Minimum USMLE Step 1 Score Requirement: No limits set
Minimum USMLE Step 2 Score Requirement: No limits set
Attempts on any step: Must pass on the first attempt
CS required at time of application: Yes including ECFMG certificate
USCE Requirement: 2-3 months (Canadian or European rotations are accepted)
Cut-Off time since graduation: 3 years
Program offers couple match: Yes
Visas Sponsored or accepted: J1 visa

New Jersey

Cooper Medical School of Rowan University/Cooper University Hospital Obstetrics and Gynecology Residency Program

Specialty: Obstetrics and Gynecology OB GYN Residency
Program name: Cooper Medical School of Rowan University/Cooper University Hospital Program
Program code: 220-33-11-162
NRMP Code: 1380220C0
Program type: University-based
State: New Jersey
Address: Cooper Hospital-University Medical Centre
       3 Cooper Plaza, Camden, NJ 08103
Phone: (856) 342-2965
Fax: (856) 365-1967
Percentage of IMGs in the program: 25%
Minimum USMLE Step 1 Score Requirement: No limits set
Minimum USMLE Step 2 Score Requirement: No limits set
Attempts on any step: No limits set
CS required at time of application: Yes including ECFMG certificate
USCE Requirement: None
Cut-Off time since graduation: 5 years
Program offers couple match: Yes

Visas Sponsored or accepted: J1 visa

Monmouth Medical Center Obstetrics and Gynecology Residency Program

Specialty: Obstetrics and Gynecology OB GYN Residency
Program name: Monmouth Medical Center Program
Program code: 220-33-11-164
State: New Jersey
Address: Monmouth Medical Center
　　　　　300 Second Ave, Long Branch, NJ 07740
Phone: (732) 923-6795
Fax: (732) 923-6793
Percentage of IMGs in the program: 80%
Minimum USMLE Step 1 Score Requirement: No limits set
Minimum USMLE Step 2 Score Requirement: No limits set
Attempts on any step: Must pass maximum on the 3rd attempt
CS required at time of application: No
USCE Requirement: None
Cut-Off time since graduation: No limits set
Program offers couple match: No
Visas Sponsored or accepted: No visa

St Barnabas Medical Center Obstetrics and Gynecology Residency Program

Specialty: Obstetrics and Gynecology OB GYN Residency
Program name: St Barnabas Medical Center Program
Program code: 220-33-12-163
NRMP Code: 1396220C0
Program type: Community-based university affiliated hospital
State: New Jersey
Address: St Barnabas Medical Center
94 Old Short Hills Rd, Livingston, NJ 07039
Phone: (973) 322-5281
Fax: (973) 533-4492
Percentage of IMGs in the program: 50%
Minimum USMLE Step 1 Score Requirement: No limits set
Minimum USMLE Step 2 Score Requirement: No limits set
Attempts on any step: No limits set
CS required at time of application: No
USCE Requirement: Yes
Cut-Off time since graduation: No limits set
Program offers couple match: Yes
Visas Sponsored or accepted: J1 visa

Jersey Shore University Medical Center Obstetrics and Gynecology Residency Program

Specialty: Obstetrics and Gynecology OB GYN Residency
Program name: Jersey Shore University Medical Center Program
Program code: 220-33-12-165
NRMP Code: 1395220C0
Program type: Community-based university affiliated hospital
State: New Jersey
Address: Jersey Shore University Medical Center

      1945 State Rte 33, Neptune, NJ 07754
Phone: (732) 776-3790
Fax: (732) 776-4525
Percentage of IMGs in the program: 40%
Minimum USMLE Step 1 Score Requirement: No limits set
Minimum USMLE Step 2 Score Requirement: No limits set
Attempts on any step: Must pass on the first attempt
CS required at time of application: Yes including ECFMG certificate
USCE Requirement: None
Cut-Off time since graduation: No limits set
Program offers couple match: Yes
Visas Sponsored or accepted: No visa

Saint Peter's University Hospital/Rutgers Robert Wood Johnson Medical School Obstetrics and Gynecology Residency Program

Specialty: Obstetrics and Gynecology OB GYN Residency
Program name: Saint Peter's University Hospital/Rutgers Robert Wood Johnson Medical School Program
Program code: 220-33-12-362
NRMP Code: 3211220C0
Program type: Community-based university affiliated hospital
State: New Jersey
Address: St Peter's University Hospital
           254 Easton Ave, New Brunswick, NJ 08901
Phone: (732) 565-5415
Fax: (732) 342-8479
Percentage of IMGs in the program: 60%
Minimum USMLE Step 1 Score Requirement: No limits set
Minimum USMLE Step 2 Score Requirement: No limits set
Attempts on any step: No limits set
CS required at time of application: Yes including ECFMG certificate

USCE Requirement: None
Cut-Off time since graduation: No limits set
Program offers couple match: Yes
Visas Sponsored or accepted: J1 visa

Rutgers Robert Wood Johnson Medical School Obstetrics and Gynecology Residency Program

Specialty: Obstetrics and Gynecology OB GYN Residency
Program name: Rutgers Robert Wood Johnson Medical School Program
Program code: 220-33-21-167
NRMP Code: 2918220C0
Program type: University-based
State: New Jersey
Address: Rutgers Robert Wood Johnson Medical School
            125 Paterson St, New Brunswick, NJ 08901
Phone: (732) 235-6375
Fax: (732) 235-9855
Percentage of IMGs in the program: 15%
Minimum USMLE Step 1 Score Requirement: No limits set
Minimum USMLE Step 2 Score Requirement: No limits set
Attempts on any step: No limits set

CS required at time of application: Yes
including ECFMG certificate
USCE Requirement: None
Cut-Off time since graduation: No limits set
Program offers couple match: Yes
Visas Sponsored or accepted: J1 visa

Newark Beth Israel Medical Center Obstetrics and Gynecology Residency Program

Specialty: Obstetrics and Gynecology OB GYN Residency
Program name: Newark Beth Israel Medical Center Program
Program code: 220-33-21-321
NRMP Code: 1397220P0, 1397220C0
Program type: Community-based
State: New Jersey
Address: Newark Beth Israel Medical Center
201 Lyons Ave, Newark, NJ 07112-2027
Phone: (973) 926-4882
Fax: (973) 923-7497
Percentage of IMGs in the program: 50%
Minimum USMLE Step 1 Score Requirement: No limits set

Minimum USMLE Step 2 Score Requirement: No limits set
Attempts on any step: Must pass on the first attempt
CS required at time of application: Yes including ECFMG certificate
USCE Requirement: Yes
Cut-Off time since graduation: 5 years
Program offers couple match: No
Visas Sponsored or accepted: No visa

New York Medical College at St Joseph's Regional Medical Center Obstetrics and Gynecology Residency Program

Specialty: Obstetrics and Gynecology OB GYN Residency
Program name: New York Medical College at St Joseph's Regional Medical Center Program
Program code: 220-33-21-323
NRMP Code: 1406220C0
Program type: Community-based university affiliated hospital
State: New Jersey
Address: St Joseph's Regional Medical Center
703 Main St, Paterson, NJ 07503
Phone: (973) 754-2726
Fax: (973) 754-2725

Percentage of IMGs in the program: 90%
Minimum USMLE Step 1 Score Requirement: No limits set
Minimum USMLE Step 2 Score Requirement: No limits set
Attempts on any step: Must pass on the first attempt
CS required at time of application: Yes including ECFMG certificate
USCE Requirement: None
Cut-Off time since graduation: 5 years
Program offers couple match: Yes
Visas Sponsored or accepted: J1 visa

Newark Beth Israel Medical Center (Jersey City) Obstetrics and Gynecology Residency Program

Specialty: Obstetrics and Gynecology OB GYN Residency
Program name: Newark Beth Israel Medical Center (Jersey City) Program
Program code: 220-33-21-324
NRMP Code: 1390220C0
Program type: Community-based
State: New Jersey
Address: Jersey City Medical Center
           355 Grand St, Jersey City, NJ 07302
Phone: (201) 915-2462
Fax: (201) 915-2481

Percentage of IMGs in the program: 60%
Minimum USMLE Step 1 Score Requirement: No limits set
Minimum USMLE Step 2 Score Requirement: No limits set
Attempts on any step: Must pass maximum on the 2nd attempt
CS required at time of application: Yes including ECFMG certificate
USCE Requirement: None
Cut-Off time since graduation: 7 years
Program offers couple match: Yes
Visas Sponsored or accepted: J1 visa

Rutgers New Jersey Medical School Obstetrics and Gynecology Residency Program

Specialty: Obstetrics and Gynecology OB GYN Residency
Program name: Rutgers New Jersey Medical School Program
Program code: 220-33-31-166
NRMP Code: 1398220C0,
Program type: University-based
State: New Jersey
Address: Rutgers New Jersey Medical School
185 S Orange Ave, Newark, NJ 07103-2714
Phone: (973) 972-5266

Fax: (973) 972-4574
Percentage of IMGs in the program: 30%
Minimum USMLE Step 1 Score Requirement: No limits set
Minimum USMLE Step 2 Score Requirement: No limits set
Attempts on any step: No limits set
CS required at time of application: Yes including ECFMG certificate
USCE Requirement: None
Cut-Off time since graduation: No limits set
Program offers couple match: No
Visas Sponsored or accepted: J1 visa

Atlantic Health (Morristown) Obstetrics and Gynecology Residency Program

Specialty: Obstetrics and Gynecology OB GYN Residency
Program name: Atlantic Health (Morristown) Program
Program code: 220-33-31-365
NRMP Code:
Program type:
State: New Jersey
Address: Morristown Medical Center
        100 Madison Ave, Morristown, NJ 07962-1956
Phone: (973) 971-6279

Fax: (973) 290-7054
Percentage of IMGs in the program: 50%
Minimum USMLE Step 1 Score Requirement: 220
Minimum USMLE Step 2 Score Requirement: 220
Attempts on any step: Must pass on the first attempt
CS required at time of application: Yes including ECFMG certificate
USCE Requirement: None
Cut-Off time since graduation: 5 years
Program offers couple match: No
Visas Sponsored or accepted: J1 visa

New Mexico

University of New Mexico Obstetrics and Gynecology Residency Program

Specialty: Obstetrics and Gynecology OB GYN Residency
Program name: University of New Mexico Program
Program code: 220-34-21-169
NRMP Code: 1962220C0

Program type: University-based
State: New Mexico
Address: University of New Mexico Health Science Center
        1 University of New Mexico, Albuquerque, NM 87131-0001
Phone: (505) 272-6883
Fax: (505) 272-3918
Percentage of IMGs in the program: 5%
Minimum USMLE Step 1 Score Requirement: 225
Minimum USMLE Step 2 Score Requirement: 225
Attempts on any step: No limits set
CS required at time of application: Yes including ECFMG certificate
USCE Requirement: None
Cut-Off time since graduation: No limits set
Program offers couple match: Yes
Visas Sponsored or accepted: J1 visa

New York

Icahn School of Medicine at Mount Sinai (Beth Israel) Obstetrics and Gynecology Residency Program

Specialty: Obstetrics and Gynecology
Program name: Icahn School of Medicine at Mount Sinai (Beth Israel) Program
Program code: 220-35-11-179
NRMP Code: 1470220C0
Program type: Community-based university affiliated hospital
State: New York
Address: Beth Israel Medical Center
　　　　　　350 E 17th St, New York, NY 10003
Phone: (212) 420-4548
Fax: (212) 420-2980
Percentage of IMGs in the program: 10%
Minimum USMLE Step 1 Score Requirement: 220
Minimum USMLE Step 2 Score Requirement: 220
Attempts on any step: Must pass on first attempt
CS required at time of application: Yes including ECFMG certificate
USCE Requirement: Yes however 1-2 years OBGYN experience outside the states is also considered
Cut-Off time since graduation: No limits set
Program offers couple match: Yes

Visas Sponsored or accepted: J1 visa and H1b visa

Bronx-Lebanon Hospital Center Obstetrics and Gynecology Residency Program

Specialty: Obstetrics and Gynecology
Program name: Bronx-Lebanon Hospital Center Program
Program code: 220-35-11-180
State: New York
Address: Bronx-Lebanon Hospital Center
1650 Grand Concourse Ave, Bronx, NY 10457
Phone: (718) 239-8384
Fax: (718) 239-8360
Percentage of IMGs in the program: 70%
Minimum USMLE Step 1 Score Requirement: 205
Minimum USMLE Step 2 Score Requirement: 205
Attempts on any step: No limits set
CS required at time of application: Yes including ECFMG certificate
USCE Requirement: None
Cut-Off time since graduation: No limits set
Program offers couple match: Yes
Visas Sponsored or accepted: J1 visa and H1b visa

Flushing Hospital Medical Center Obstetrics and Gynecology Residency Program

Specialty: Obstetrics and Gynecology
Program name: Flushing Hospital Medical Center Program
Program code: 220-35-11-184
NRMP Code: 1445220P0, 1445220C0
Program type: Community-based
State: New York
Address: Flushing Hospital Medical Center
4500 Parsons Blvd, Flushing, NY 11355
Phone: (718) 670-5440
Fax: (718) 670-5780
Percentage of IMGs in the program: 100%
Minimum USMLE Step 1 Score Requirement: No limits set
Minimum USMLE Step 2 Score Requirement: No limits set
Attempts on any step: No limits set
CS required at time of application: Yes including ECFMG certificate
USCE Requirement: None
Cut-Off time since graduation: No limits set
Program offers couple match: No
Visas Sponsored or accepted: J1 visa

NSLIJ/Hofstra North Shore-LIJ School of Medicine at Lenox Hill Hospital Obstetrics and Gynecology Residency Program

Specialty: Obstetrics and Gynecology
Program name: NSLIJ/Hofstra North Shore-LIJ School of Medicine at Lenox Hill Hospital Program
Program code: 220-35-11-188
NRMP Code: 1483220C0
Program type: Community-based University affiliated hospital
State: New York
Address: Lenox Hill Hospital
130 E 77th St, New York, NY 10021-1883
Phone: (212) 434-2160
Fax: (212) 434-2180
Percentage of IMGs in the program: 20%
Minimum USMLE Step 1 Score Requirement: No limits set
Minimum USMLE Step 2 Score Requirement: No limits set
Attempts on any step: No limits set
CS required at time of application: No
USCE Requirement: None
Cut-Off time since graduation: No limits set
Program offers couple match: Yes

Visas Sponsored or accepted: J1 visa and H1b
visa

Lutheran Medical Center Obstetrics and Gynecology Residency Program

Specialty: Obstetrics and Gynecology
Program name: Lutheran Medical Center
Program
Program code: 220-35-11-191
NRMP Code: 1430220C0
Program type: Community-based University
affiliated hospital
State: New York
Address: Lutheran Medical Center
          150 55th St, Brooklyn, NY 11220
Phone: (718) 630-6834
Fax: (718) 630-7865
Percentage of IMGs in the program: 15%
Minimum USMLE Step 1 Score Requirement:
210
Minimum USMLE Step 2 Score Requirement:
210
Attempts on any step: No limits set
CS required at time of application: Yes
including ECFMG certificate
USCE Requirement: None
Cut-Off time since graduation: No limits set
Program offers couple match: Yes

Visas Sponsored or accepted: J1 visa and H1b visa

Icahn School of Medicine at Mount Sinai/St Luke's-Roosevelt Hospital Center Obstetrics and Gynecology Residency Program

Specialty: Obstetrics and Gynecology
Program name: Icahn School of Medicine at Mount Sinai/St Luke's-Roosevelt Hospital Center Program
Program code: 220-35-11-204
NRMP Code: 2070220C0
Program type: Community-based university affiliated hospital
State: New York
Address: St Lukes-Roosevelt Hospital Center
1000 Tenth Ave, New York, NY 10019
Phone: (212) 523-8366
Fax: (212) 523-8066
Percentage of IMGs in the program: 10% (variable)
Minimum USMLE Step 1 Score Requirement: 230
Minimum USMLE Step 2 Score Requirement: 220
Attempts on any step: Must pass maximum on the 2nd attempt

CS required at time of application: Yes including ECFMG certificate
USCE Requirement: None
Cut-Off time since graduation: No limits set
Program offers couple match: Yes
Visas Sponsored or accepted: J1 visa and H1b visa

Staten Island University Hospital Obstetrics and Gynecology Residency Program

Specialty: Obstetrics and Gynecology
Program name: Staten Island University Hospital Program
Program code: 220-35-11-207
NRMP Code: 1515220C0
Program type: Community-based University affiliated hospital
State: New York
Address: Staten Island University Hospital
475 Seaview Ave, Staten Island, NY 10305
Phone: (718) 226-8074
Fax: (718) 226-6873
Percentage of IMGs in the program: 60%
Minimum USMLE Step 1 Score Requirement: No limits set
Minimum USMLE Step 2 Score Requirement: No limits set

Attempts on any step: No limits set
CS required at time of application: Yes including ECFMG certificate
USCE Requirement: None
Cut-Off time since graduation: No limits set
Program offers couple match: Yes
Visas Sponsored or accepted: J1 visa and H1b visa

Winthrop-University Hospital Obstetrics and Gynecology Residency Program

Specialty: Obstetrics and Gynecology
Program name: Winthrop-University Hospital Program
Program code: 220-35-12-176
NRMP Code: 1455220C0
Program type: Community-based University affiliated hospital
State: New York
Address: Winthrop-University Hospital
259 First St, Mineola, NY 11501
Phone: (516) 663-2264
Fax: (516) 742-7821
Percentage of IMGs in the program: 0%
Minimum USMLE Step 1 Score Requirement: 200
Minimum USMLE Step 2 Score Requirement: 215

Attempts on any step: Must pass on first attempt
CS required at time of application: Yes including ECFMG certificate
USCE Requirement: None
Cut-Off time since graduation: 3 years
Program offers couple match: Yes
Visas Sponsored or accepted: J1 visa and H1b visa

Brooklyn Hospital Center Obstetrics and Gynecology Residency Program

Specialty: Obstetrics and Gynecology
Program name: Brooklyn Hospital Center Program
Program code: 220-35-12-182
NRMP Code: 1420220C0
Program type: Community-based university affiliated hospital
State: New York
Address: Brooklyn Hospital Center
121 DeKalb Ave, Brooklyn, NY 11201
Phone: (718) 250-8322
Fax: (718) 250-8881
Percentage of IMGs in the program: 100%
Minimum USMLE Step 1 Score Requirement: No limits set
Minimum USMLE Step 2 Score Requirement: No limits set

Attempts on any step: No limits set
CS required at time of application: Yes
including ECFMG certificate
USCE Requirement: None
Cut-Off time since graduation: No limits set
Program offers couple match: Yes
Visas Sponsored or accepted: J1 visa and H1b
visa

Richmond University Medical Center Obstetrics and Gynecology Residency Program

Specialty: Obstetrics and Gynecology
Program name: Richmond University Medical
Center Program
Program code: 220-35-12-206
State: New York
Address: Richmond University Medical Center
            355 Bard Ave, Staten Island, NY 10310
Phone: (718) 818-4273
Fax: (718) 818-3943
Percentage of IMGs in the program: 50%
Minimum USMLE Step 1 Score Requirement:
No limits set
Minimum USMLE Step 2 Score Requirement:
No limits set
Attempts on any step: No limits set
CS required at time of application: Yes
including ECFMG certificate

USCE Requirement: None
Cut-Off time since graduation: No limits set
Program offers couple match: Yes
Visas Sponsored or accepted: J1 visa and H1b visa

Albany Medical Center Obstetrics and Gynecology Residency Program

Specialty: Obstetrics and Gynecology
Program name: Albany Medical Center Program
Program code: 220-35-21-170
NRMP Code: 1414220C0
Program type: University-based
State: New York
Address: Albany Medical Center
          16 New Scotland Ave, Albany, NY 12208
Phone: (518) 264-5026
Fax: (518) 262-2675
Percentage of IMGs in the program: 0%
Minimum USMLE Step 1 Score Requirement: No limits set
Minimum USMLE Step 2 Score Requirement: No limits set
Attempts on any step: Must pass on first attempt
CS required at time of application: Yes including ECFMG certificate

USCE Requirement: None
Cut-Off time since graduation: 2 years
Program offers couple match: Yes
Visas Sponsored or accepted: J1 visa

University at Buffalo (Sisters of Charity) Obstetrics and Gynecology Residency Program

Specialty: Obstetrics and Gynecology
Program name: University at Buffalo (Sisters of Charity) Program
Program code: 220-35-21-171
State: New York
Address: Sisters of Charity Hospital
2157 Main St, Buffalo, NY 14214
Phone: (716) 862-1589
Fax: (716) 862-1881
Percentage of IMGs in the program: 20%
Minimum USMLE Step 1 Score Requirement: No limits set
Minimum USMLE Step 2 Score Requirement: No limits set
Attempts on any step: No limits set
CS required at time of application: No
USCE Requirement: None
Cut-Off time since graduation: No limits set
Program offers couple match: Yes
Visas Sponsored or accepted: No visa

University at Buffalo Obstetrics and Gynecology Residency Program

Specialty: Obstetrics and Gynecology
Program name: University at Buffalo Program
Program code: 220-35-21-172
NRMP Code: 3099220C0
Program type: University-based
State: New York
Address: Women and Children's Hospital of Buffalo

       219 Bryant St, Buffalo, NY 14222
Phone: (716) 878-7750
Fax: (716) 888-3833
Percentage of IMGs in the program: 50%
Minimum USMLE Step 1 Score Requirement: No limits set
Minimum USMLE Step 2 Score Requirement: No limits set
Attempts on any step: No limits set
CS required at time of application: No
USCE Requirement: None
Cut-Off time since graduation: No limits set
Program offers couple match: Yes
Visas Sponsored or accepted: J1 visa

Albert Einstein College of Medicine Obstetrics and Gynecology Residency Program

Specialty: Obstetrics and Gynecology
Program name: Albert Einstein College of Medicine Program
Program code: 220-35-21-178
NRMP Code: 3153220C0
Program type: University-based
State: New York
Address: Albert Einstein College of Medicine
1300 Morris Park Ave, Bronx, NY 10461
Phone: (718) 430-4031
Fax: (718) 430-8774
Percentage of IMGs in the program: 20%
Minimum USMLE Step 1 Score Requirement: No limits set
Minimum USMLE Step 2 Score Requirement: No limits set
Attempts on any step: Preferably no failures
CS required at time of application: No
USCE Requirement: None
Cut-Off time since graduation: No limits set
Program offers couple match: Yes
Visas Sponsored or accepted: J1 visa and H1b

Jamaica Hospital Medical Center Obstetrics and Gynecology Residency Program

Specialty: Obstetrics and Gynecology
Program name: Jamaica Hospital Medical Center Program
Program code: 220-35-21-186
NRMP Code: 1449220C0, 1449220P0
Program type: Community-based
State: New York
Address: Jamaica Hospital Medical Center
8900 Van Wyck Expwy, Jamaica, NY 11418
Phone: (718) 206-6808
Fax: (718) 206-6829
Percentage of IMGs in the program: 100%
Minimum USMLE Step 1 Score Requirement: No limits set
Minimum USMLE Step 2 Score Requirement: No limits set
Attempts on any step: Prefer passage on first attempt but not strict
CS required at time of application: Yes including ECFMG certificate
USCE Requirement: Yes at least 1-2 months within the last 2 years
Cut-Off time since graduation: 5 years
Program offers couple match: Yes
Visas Sponsored or accepted: J1 visa

NSLIJHS/Hofstra North Shore-LIJ School of Medicine Obstetrics and Gynecology Residency Program

Specialty: Obstetrics and Gynecology
Program name: NSLIJHS/Hofstra North Shore-LIJ School of Medicine Program
Program code: 220-35-21-190
NRMP Code: 1700220C0, 1700220P0
Program type: University-based
State: New York
Address: North Shore University Hospital
300 Community Dr, Manhasset, NY 11030
Phone: (516) 562-4429
Fax: (516) 562-1299
Percentage of IMGs in the program: 0%
Minimum USMLE Step 1 Score Requirement: No limits set
Minimum USMLE Step 2 Score Requirement: No limits set
Attempts on any step: No limits set
CS required at time of application: No
USCE Requirement: None
Cut-Off time since graduation: No limits set
Program offers couple match: Yes
Visas Sponsored or accepted: J1 visa and H1b visa

Icahn School of Medicine at Mount Sinai Obstetrics and Gynecology Residency Program

Specialty: Obstetrics and Gynecology
Program name: Icahn School of Medicine at Mount Sinai Program
Program code: 220-35-21-196
NRMP Code: 1490220C0, 1490220P0
Program type: University-based
State: New York
Address: Mount Sinai Medical Center
One Gustave L Levy Pl, New York, NY 10029
Phone: (212) 241-8578
Fax: (212) 241-3833
Percentage of IMGs in the program: 15% (Variable)
Minimum USMLE Step 1 Score Requirement: 200
Minimum USMLE Step 2 Score Requirement: 205
Attempts on any step: Must pass on first attempt
CS required at time of application: Yes including ECFMG certificate
USCE Requirement: Yes but 1-2 years experience outside the US is considered
Cut-Off time since graduation: No limits set

Program offers couple match: Yes
Visas Sponsored or accepted: J1 visa and H1b visa

New York Presbyterian Hospital (Cornell Campus) Obstetrics and Gynecology Residency Program

Specialty: Obstetrics and Gynecology
Program name: New York Presbyterian Hospital (Cornell Campus) Program
Program code: 220-35-21-197
NRMP Code: 1492220C0, 1492220P0
Program type: University-based
State: New York
Address: New York Presbyterian Hospital-Cornell

       525 E 68th St, New York, NY 10065
Phone: (212) 746-3058
Fax: (212) 746-8490
Percentage of IMGs in the program: 5% (Variable)
Minimum USMLE Step 1 Score Requirement: No limits set
Minimum USMLE Step 2 Score Requirement: No limits set
Attempts on any step: No limits set
CS required at time of application: Yes including ECFMG certificate
USCE Requirement: None

Cut-Off time since graduation: No limits set
Program offers couple match: Yes
Visas Sponsored or accepted: J1 visa

New York Medical College at Westchester Medical Center Obstetrics and Gynecology Residency Program

Specialty: Obstetrics and Gynecology
Program name: New York Medical College at Westchester Medical Center Program
Program code: 220-35-21-199
NRMP Code: 1443220P0, 1443220C0
Program type: University-based
State: New York
Address: Metropolitan Hospital Center
1901 First Ave, New York, NY 10029
Phone: (212) 423-6796   Ext: 6796
Fax: (212) 423-8121
Percentage of IMGs in the program: 0%
(Occasionally one)
Minimum USMLE Step 1 Score Requirement:
No limits set
Minimum USMLE Step 2 Score Requirement:
No limits set
Attempts on any step: No limits set
CS required at time of application: Yes
including ECFMG certificate
USCE Requirement: None

Cut-Off time since graduation: No limits set
Program offers couple match: Yes
Visas Sponsored or accepted: No visa

New York University School of Medicine Obstetrics and Gynecology Residency Program

Specialty: Obstetrics and Gynecology
Program name: New York University School of Medicine Program
Program code: 220-35-21-200
NRMP Code: 2978220C0
Program type: University-based
State: New York
Address: New York University Medical Center
550 First Ave, New York, NY 10016
Phone: (212) 263-6453
Fax: (212) 263-8251
Percentage of IMGs in the program: 8%
Minimum USMLE Step 1 Score Requirement: No limits set
Minimum USMLE Step 2 Score Requirement: No limits set
Attempts on any step: No limits set
CS required at time of application: Yes including ECFMG certificate
USCE Requirement: None
Cut-Off time since graduation: No limits set
Program offers couple match: Yes

Visas Sponsored or accepted: J1 visa and H1b visa

New York Presbyterian Hospital (Columbia Campus) Obstetrics and Gynecology Residency Program

Specialty: Obstetrics and Gynecology
Program name: New York Presbyterian Hospital (Columbia Campus) Program
Program code: 220-35-21-201
NRMP Code: 1495220C0
Program type: University-based
State: New York
Address: New York Presbyterian Hospital-Columbia
          622 W 168th St, New York, NY 10032
Phone: (212) 305-2376
Fax: (212) 305-4672
Percentage of IMGs in the program: 0%
Minimum USMLE Step 1 Score Requirement: No limits set
Minimum USMLE Step 2 Score Requirement: No limits set
Attempts on any step: No limits set
CS required at time of application: No
USCE Requirement: None
Cut-Off time since graduation: No limits set
Program offers couple match: Yes

SUNY Health Science Center at Brooklyn Obstetrics and Gynecology Residency Program

Specialty: Obstetrics and Gynecology
Program name: SUNY Health Science Center at Brooklyn Program
Program code: 220-35-21-208
State: New York
Address: SUNY Downstate Medical Center
          450 Clarkson Ave, Brooklyn, NY 11203-2098
Phone: (718) 270-3320
Fax: (718) 270-4122
Percentage of IMGs in the program: 40%
Minimum USMLE Step 1 Score Requirement: No limits set
Minimum USMLE Step 2 Score Requirement: No limits set
Attempts on any step: No limits set
CS required at time of application: No
USCE Requirement: None
Cut-Off time since graduation: No limits set
Program offers couple match: Yes
Visas Sponsored or accepted: J1 visa and H1b visa

University of Rochester Obstetrics and Gynecology Residency Program

Specialty: Obstetrics and Gynecology
Program name: University of Rochester Program
Program code: 220-35-21-213
NRMP Code: 1511220C0
Program type: University-based
State: New York
Address: University of Rochester Medical Center
      601 Elmwood Ave Rochester, NY 14642-8668
Phone: (585) 275-3733
Fax: (585) 756-4967
Percentage of IMGs in the program: 0% (Occasionally one)
Minimum USMLE Step 1 Score Requirement: No limits set
Minimum USMLE Step 2 Score Requirement: No limits set
Attempts on any step: No limits set
CS required at time of application: Yes including ECFMG certificate
USCE Requirement: None
Cut-Off time since graduation: 5 years
Program offers couple match: Yes
Visas Sponsored or accepted: J1 visa

SUNY Upstate Medical University Obstetrics and Gynecology Residency Program

Specialty: Obstetrics and Gynecology
Program name: SUNY Upstate Medical University Program
Program code: 220-35-21-215
NRMP Code: 1516220C0
Program type: University-based
State: New York
Address: SUNY Upstate Medical Center
          750 E Adams St, Syracuse, NY 13210
Phone: (315) 464-5692
Percentage of IMGs in the program: 0%-40% (Varies from year to year)
Minimum USMLE Step 1 Score Requirement: No limits set
Minimum USMLE Step 2 Score Requirement: No limits set
Attempts on any step: No limits set
CS required at time of application: Yes including ECFMG certificate
USCE Requirement: None
Cut-Off time since graduation: No limits set but recent clinical experience required
Program offers couple match: Yes
Visas Sponsored or accepted: J1 visa

SUNY at Stony Brook Obstetrics and Gynecology Residency Program

Specialty: Obstetrics and Gynecology
Program name: SUNY at Stony Brook Program
Program code: 220-35-21-316
NRMP Code: 2919220C0
Program type: University-based
State: New York
Address: SUNY Stony Brook University
         Health Science Center T-9, Stony
Brook, NY 11794-8091
Phone: (631) 444-2739
Fax: (631) 444-8954
Percentage of IMGs in the program: 0%
Minimum USMLE Step 1 Score Requirement:
No limits set
Minimum USMLE Step 2 Score Requirement:
No limits set
Attempts on any step: No limits set
CS required at time of application: Yes
including ECFMG certificate
USCE Requirement: None
Cut-Off time since graduation: No limits set
Program offers couple match: Yes
Visas Sponsored or accepted: J1 visa

Lincoln Medical and Mental Health Center Obstetrics and Gynecology Residency Program

Specialty: Obstetrics and Gynecology
Program name: Lincoln Medical and Mental Health Center Program
Program code: 220-35-21-326
State: New York
Address: Lincoln Medical and Mental Health Center

234 E 149th St, Bronx, NY 10451
Phone: (718) 579-5830
Fax: (718) 579-4699
Percentage of IMGs in the program: 40%
Minimum USMLE Step 1 Score Requirement: 205
Minimum USMLE Step 2 Score Requirement: 205
Attempts on any step: No limits set
CS required at time of application: No
USCE Requirement: None
Cut-Off time since graduation: 4 years
Program offers couple match: No
Visas Sponsored or accepted: J1 visa and H1b visa

Icahn School of Medicine at Mount Sinai (Jamaica) Obstetrics and Gynecology Residency Program

Specialty: Obstetrics and Gynecology
Program name: Icahn School of Medicine at Mount Sinai (Jamaica) Program
Program code: 220-35-21-342
NRMP Code: 1489220C0
Program type: Community-based university affiliated hospital
State: New York
Address: Queens Hospital Center
        82-68 164th St, Jamaica, NY 11432
Phone: (718) 883-4037
Fax: (718) 883-6129
Percentage of IMGs in the program: 80%
Minimum USMLE Step 1 Score Requirement: No limits set
Minimum USMLE Step 2 Score Requirement: No limits set
Attempts on any step: No limits set
CS required at time of application: Yes including ECFMG certificate
USCE Requirement: None
Cut-Off time since graduation: No limits set
Program offers couple match: Yes
Visas Sponsored or accepted: J1 visa and H1b visa

Nassau University Medical Center Obstetrics and Gynecology Residency Program

Specialty: Obstetrics and Gynecology
Program name: Nassau University Medical Center Program
Program code: 220-35-31-174
State: New York
Address: Nassau University Medical Center
        2201 Hempstead Trnpk, East Meadow, NY 11554
Phone: (516) 296-2830
Fax: (516) 572-3124
Percentage of IMGs in the program: 50%
Minimum USMLE Step 1 Score Requirement: No limits set
Minimum USMLE Step 2 Score Requirement: No limits set
Attempts on any step: No limits set
CS required at time of application: Yes including ECFMG certificate
USCE Requirement: None
Cut-Off time since graduation: 5 years
Program offers couple match: Yes
Visas Sponsored or accepted: J1 visa

Maimonides Medical Center Obstetrics and Gynecology Residency Program

Specialty: Obstetrics and Gynecology
Program name: Maimonides Medical Center Program
Program code: 220-35-31-192
NRMP Code: 1428220C0
Program type: Community-based
State: New York
Address: Maimonides Medical Center
4802 Tenth Ave, Brooklyn, NY 11219
Phone: (718) 283-6078
Fax: (718) 283-8468
Percentage of IMGs in the program: 60%
Minimum USMLE Step 1 Score Requirement: No limits set
Minimum USMLE Step 2 Score Requirement: No limits set
Attempts on any step: Must pass on first attempt
CS required at time of application: Yes including ECFMG certificate
USCE Requirement: None
Cut-Off time since graduation: No limits set
Program offers couple match: Yes
Visas Sponsored or accepted: J1 visa and H1b visa

New York Methodist Hospital Obstetrics and Gynecology Residency Program

Specialty: Obstetrics and Gynecology
Program name: New York Methodist Hospital Program
Program code: 220-35-31-339
NRMP Code: 1429220C0
Program type: Community-based university affiliated hospital
State: New York
Address: New York Methodist Hospital
             506 Sixth St, Brooklyn, NY 11215
Phone: (718) 780-5213
Fax: (718) 780-3079
Percentage of IMGs in the program: 50%
Minimum USMLE Step 1 Score Requirement: No limits set
Minimum USMLE Step 2 Score Requirement: No limits set
Attempts on any step: No limits set
CS required at time of application: Yes including ECFMG certificate
USCE Requirement: None
Cut-Off time since graduation: No limits set
Program offers couple match: Yes
Visas Sponsored or accepted: No visa

Rochester General Hospital Obstetrics and Gynecology Residency Program

Specialty: Obstetrics and Gynecology
Program name: Rochester General Hospital Program
Program code: 220-35-31-343
NRMP Code: 1509220C0
Program type: Community-based university affiliated hospital
State: New York
Address: Rochester General Hospital
        1425 Portland Ave, Rochester, NY 14621-3095
Phone: (585) 922-4683
Fax: (585) 922-3606
Percentage of IMGs in the program: 95%
Minimum USMLE Step 1 Score Requirement: No limits set
Minimum USMLE Step 2 Score Requirement: No limits set
Attempts on any step: Must pass on first attempt
CS required at time of application: Yes including ECFMG certificate
USCE Requirement: None but preferred
Cut-Off time since graduation: No limits set
Program offers couple match: Yes
Visas Sponsored or accepted: J1 visa and H1b visa

North Carolina

New Hanover Regional Medical Center Obstetrics and Gynecology Residency Program

Specialty: Obstetrics and Gynecology
Program name: New Hanover Regional Medical Center Program
Program code: 220-36-11-218
NRMP Code: 1534220P0, 1534220C0
Program type: Community-based university affiliated hospital
State: North Carolina
Address: New Hanover Regional Medical Center
2131 S 17th St, Wilmington, NC 28401
Phone: (910) 667-9237
Fax: (910) 762-2896
Percentage of IMGs in the program: 0%
Minimum USMLE Step 1 Score Requirement: 210
Minimum USMLE Step 2 Score Requirement: 210
Attempts on any step: No limits set

CS required at time of application: Yes
including ECFMG certificate
USCE Requirement: None
Cut-Off time since graduation: No limits set
Program offers couple match: Yes
Visas Sponsored or accepted: No visa

University of North Carolina Hospitals Obstetrics and Gynecology Residency Program

Specialty: Obstetrics and Gynecology
Program name: University of North Carolina
Hospitals Program
Program code: 220-36-21-216
State: North Carolina
Address: University of North Carolina Hospitals
CB#7570, Chapel Hill, NC 27514
Phone: (919) 966-5671
Fax: (919) 843-1480
Percentage of IMGs in the program: 0%
Minimum USMLE Step 1 Score Requirement:
No limits set
Minimum USMLE Step 2 Score Requirement:
No limits set
Attempts on any step: No limits set
CS required at time of application: Yes
including ECFMG certificate
USCE Requirement: None
Cut-Off time since graduation: No limits set

Program offers couple match: No
Visas Sponsored or accepted: No visa

Duke University Hospital Obstetrics and Gynecology Residency Program

Specialty: Obstetrics and Gynecology
Program name: Duke University Hospital Program
Program code: 220-36-21-219
State: North Carolina
Address: Duke University Medical Center
200 Trent Dr, Durham, NC 27710
Phone: (919) 668-2591
Fax: (919) 668-5547
Percentage of IMGs in the program: 0%
Minimum USMLE Step 1 Score Requirement: No limits set
Minimum USMLE Step 2 Score Requirement: No limits set
Attempts on any step: No limits set
CS required at time of application: Yes including ECFMG certificate
USCE Requirement: None
Cut-Off time since graduation: No limits set
Program offers couple match: Yes
Visas Sponsored or accepted: J1 visa and H1b visa

Vidant Medical Center/East Carolina University Obstetrics and Gynecology Residency Program

Specialty: Obstetrics and Gynecology
Program name: Vidant Medical Center/East Carolina University Program
Program code: 220-36-21-220
NRMP Code: 3057220C0
Program type: University-based
State: North Carolina
Address: Vidant Medical Center ECU
600 Moye Blvd, Greenville, NC 27834
Phone: (252) 744-4669
Fax: (252) 744-5329
Percentage of IMGs in the program: 10%
Minimum USMLE Step 1 Score Requirement: No limits set
Minimum USMLE Step 2 Score Requirement: No limits set
Attempts on any step: No limits set
CS required at time of application: No
USCE Requirement: None
Cut-Off time since graduation: No limits set
Program offers couple match: Yes
Visas Sponsored or accepted: J1 visa

Wake Forest University School of Medicine Obstetrics and Gynecology Residency Program

Specialty: Obstetrics and Gynecology
Program name: Wake Forest University School of Medicine Program
Program code: 220-36-21-221
NRMP Code: 1537220C0
Program type: University-based
State: North Carolina
Address: Wake Forest Baptist Medical Center
          Medical Center Blvd, Winston-Salem,
NC 27157-1066
Phone: (336) 716-4615
Fax: (336) 716-6937
Percentage of IMGs in the program: 5%
Minimum USMLE Step 1 Score Requirement:
No limits set
Minimum USMLE Step 2 Score Requirement:
No limits set
Attempts on any step: No limits set
CS required at time of application: No
USCE Requirement: None
Cut-Off time since graduation: No limits set
Program offers couple match: Yes
Visas Sponsored or accepted: No visa

Mountain Area Health Education Center Obstetrics and Gynecology Residency Program

Specialty: Obstetrics and Gynecology
Program name: Mountain Area Health Education Center Program
Program code: 220-36-21-340
NRMP Code: 3023220C0
Program type: Community-based
State: North Carolina
Address: Mountain Area Health Education Center

119 Hendersonville Rd, Asheville, NC 28803
Phone: (828) 771-5537
Fax: (828) 407-2662
Percentage of IMGs in the program: 0%
Minimum USMLE Step 1 Score Requirement: No limits set
Minimum USMLE Step 2 Score Requirement: No limits set
Attempts on any step: Must pass maximum on the 3rd attempt
CS required at time of application: Yes including ECFMG certificate
USCE Requirement: 1-2 months
Cut-Off time since graduation: No limits set
Program offers couple match: Yes
Visas Sponsored or accepted: J1 visa

Carolinas Medical Center Obstetrics and Gynecology Residency Program

Specialty: Obstetrics and Gynecology
Program name: Carolinas Medical Center Program
Program code: 220-36-31-217
NRMP Code: 1527220C0
Program type: Community-based university affiliated hospital
State: North Carolina
Address: Carolinas Medical Center
1000 Blythe Blvd, Charlotte, NC 28232-2861
Phone: (704) 355-2940
Fax: (704) 355-1941
Percentage of IMGs in the program: 0%
Minimum USMLE Step 1 Score Requirement: 220
Minimum USMLE Step 2 Score Requirement: 220
Attempts on any step: No limits set
CS required at time of application: No
USCE Requirement: None
Cut-Off time since graduation: No limits set
Program offers couple match: Yes
Visas Sponsored or accepted: J1 visa

Ohio

Akron General Medical Center/NEOMED Obstetrics and Gynecology Residency Program

Specialty: Obstetrics and Gynecology OB GYN Residency
Program name: Akron General Medical Center/NEOMED Program
Program code: 220-38-11-224
NRMP Code: 1542220C0
Program type: Community-based university affiliated hospital
State: Ohio
Address: Akron General Medical Center
1 Akron General Ave, Akron, OH 44307
Phone: (330) 344-6337
Fax: (330) 996-2912
Percentage of IMGs in the program: 0%
Minimum USMLE Step 1 Score Requirement: 210
Minimum USMLE Step 2 Score Requirement: 210
Attempts on any step: Must pass on the first attempt
CS required at time of application: Yes including ECFMG certificate
USCE Requirement: None
Cut-Off time since graduation: 2 years

Program offers couple match: Yes
Visas Sponsored or accepted: J1 visa and H1 b visa

TriHealth (Bethesda North and Good Samaritan Hospitals) Obstetrics and Gynecology Residency Program

Specialty: Obstetrics and Gynecology OB GYN Residency
Program name: TriHealth (Bethesda North and Good Samaritan Hospitals) Program
Program code: 220-38-11-228
NRMP Code: 1550220C0
Program type: Community-based
State: Ohio
Address: Good Samaritan Hospital
          375 Dixmyth Ave, Cincinnati, OH 45220
Phone: (513) 862-3400
Fax: (513) 221-5865
Percentage of IMGs in the program: 15%
Minimum USMLE Step 1 Score Requirement: 220
Minimum USMLE Step 2 Score Requirement: 220
Attempts on any step: Must pass maximum from the 2nd attempt

CS required at time of application: Yes
including ECFMG certificate
USCE Requirement: Yes
Cut-Off time since graduation: 4 years
Program offers couple match: Yes
Visas Sponsored or accepted: No visa

Ohio State University/Mount Carmel Hospital Obstetrics and Gynecology Residency Program

Specialty: Obstetrics and Gynecology OB GYN Residency
Program name: Ohio State University/Mount Carmel Hospital Program
Program code: 220-38-11-234
NRMP Code: 1566220C0
Program type: University-based
State: Ohio
Address: Ohio State University Medical Center
395 W 12th Ave, Columbus, OH 43210
Phone: (614) 293-4532
Fax: (614) 293-5877
Percentage of IMGs in the program: 0%
Minimum USMLE Step 1 Score Requirement:
No limits set
Minimum USMLE Step 2 Score Requirement:
No limits set
Attempts on any step: No limits set

CS required at time of application: Yes including ECFMG certificate
USCE Requirement: None
Cut-Off time since graduation: No limits set
Program offers couple match: Yes
Visas Sponsored or accepted: J1 visa

Summa Health System/NEOMED Obstetrics and Gynecology OB GYN Residency Program

Specialty: Obstetrics and Gynecology OB GYN Residency
Program name: Summa Health System/NEOMED Program
Program code: 220-38-21-223
NRMP Code: 1541220C0
Program type: Community-based university affiliated hospital
State: Ohio
Address: Summa Health System
525 E Market St, Akron, OH 44304
Phone: (330) 375-7459
Fax: (330) 375-7813
Percentage of IMGs in the program: 0%
Minimum USMLE Step 1 Score Requirement: 210

Minimum USMLE Step 2 Score Requirement: 210
Attempts on any step: Must pass on the first attempt
CS required at time of application: Yes including ECFMG certificate
USCE Requirement: None
Cut-Off time since graduation: 3 years
Program offers couple match: Yes
Visas Sponsored or accepted: J1 visa

Aultman Hospital/NEOMED Obstetrics and Gynecology Residency Program

Specialty: Obstetrics and Gynecology OB GYN Residency
Program name: Aultman Hospital/NEOMED Program
Program code: 220-38-21-226
NRMP Code: 1544220C0,
Program type: Community-based university affiliated hospital
State: Ohio
Address: Aultman Hospital
        2600 Sixth St SW, Canton, OH 44710-1799
Phone: (330) 994-1286
Fax: (330) 994-1296
Percentage of IMGs in the program: 25%

Minimum USMLE Step 1 Score Requirement:
No limits set
Minimum USMLE Step 2 Score Requirement:
No limits set
Attempts on any step: No limits set
CS required at time of application: No
USCE Requirement: None
Cut-Off time since graduation: No limits set
Program offers couple match: Yes
Visas Sponsored or accepted: J1 visa and H1b visa

University of Cincinnati Medical Center/College of Medicine Obstetrics and Gynecology Residency Program

Specialty: Obstetrics and Gynecology OB GYN Residency
Program name: University of Cincinnati Medical Center/College of Medicine Program
Program code: 220-38-21-229
NRMP Code: 1548220C0
Program type: University-based
State: Ohio
Address: University of Cincinnati Medical Center

231 Albert Sabin Way,
Cincinnati, OH 45267-0526
Phone: (513) 558-7653
Fax: (513) 558-6138
Percentage of IMGs in the program: 0%
**Minimum USMLE Step 1 Score
Requirement:** 220
**Minimum USMLE Step 2 Score
Requirement:** 220
Attempts on any step: No limits set
CS required at time of application: No
USCE Requirement: None
Cut-Off time since graduation: 5 years
Program offers couple match: Yes
Visas Sponsored or accepted: J1 visa

Case Western Reserve University/University Hospitals Case Medical Center Obstetrics and Gynecology Residency Program

Specialty: Obstetrics and Gynecology OB GYN Residency
Program name: Case Western Reserve University/University Hospitals Case Medical Center Program
Program code: 220-38-21-230
State: Ohio

Address: University MacDonald Women's Hospital

11100 Euclid Ave, Cleveland, OH 44106

Phone: (216) 844-8551
Fax: (216) 201-4239
Percentage of IMGs in the program: 10%
Minimum USMLE Step 1 Score Requirement: No limits set
Minimum USMLE Step 2 Score Requirement: No limits set
Attempts on any step: Must pass on the first attempt
CS required at time of application: No
USCE Requirement: None
Cut-Off time since graduation: No limits set
Program offers couple match: Yes
Visas Sponsored or accepted: J1 visa

Wright State University Obstetrics and Gynecology Residency Program

Specialty: Obstetrics and Gynecology OB GYN Residency
Program name: Wright State University Program
Program code: 220-38-21-236
State: Ohio

Address: Miami Valley Hospital
128 E Apple St, Dayton, OH 45409-2793
Phone: (937) 208-2287
Fax: (937) 222-7255
Percentage of IMGs in the program: 0%
Minimum USMLE Step 1 Score Requirement: No limits set
Minimum USMLE Step 2 Score Requirement: No limits set
Attempts on any step: No limits set
CS required at time of application: Yes including ECFMG certificate
USCE Requirement: Yes, 12 months
Cut-Off time since graduation: No limits set
Program offers couple match: Yes
Visas Sponsored or accepted: No visa

Case Western Reserve University (MetroHealth) Obstetrics and Gynecology Residency Program

Specialty: Obstetrics and Gynecology OB GYN Residency
Program name: Case Western Reserve University (MetroHealth) Program
Program code: 220-38-21-327
NRMP Code: 1553220P0, 1553220C0
Program type: University-based
State: Ohio

Address: MetroHealth Medical Center
2500 MetroHealth Dr, Cleveland, OH
44109-1998
Phone: (216) 778-5539
Fax: (216) 778-8642
Percentage of IMGs in the program: 25%
Minimum USMLE Step 1 Score Requirement:
No limits set
Minimum USMLE Step 2 Score Requirement:
No limits set
Attempts on any step: No limits set
CS required at time of application: Yes
including ECFMG certificate
USCE Requirement: Yes, 1 month
Cut-Off time since graduation: No limits set
Program offers couple match: Yes
Visas Sponsored or accepted: J1 visa and H1b
visa

Cleveland Clinic Foundation Obstetrics and Gynecology Residency Program

Specialty: Obstetrics and Gynecology OB GYN
Residency
Program name: Cleveland Clinic Foundation
Program
Program code: 220-38-21-370
NRMP Code: 1968220C0
Program type: University-based

State: Ohio
Address: Cleveland Clinic
        9500 Euclid Ave, Cleveland, OH 44195
Phone: (216) 444-4884
Fax: (216) 636-1296
Percentage of IMGs in the program: 0%
Minimum USMLE Step 1 Score Requirement: 210
Minimum USMLE Step 2 Score Requirement: 210
Attempts on any step: Must pass on the first attempt
CS required at time of application: Yes including ECFMG certificate
USCE Requirement: None
Cut-Off time since graduation: No limits set
Program offers couple match: Yes
Visas Sponsored or accepted: J1 visa and H1b visa

University of Toledo Obstetrics and Gynecology Residency Program

Specialty: Obstetrics and Gynecology OB GYN Residency
Program name: University of Toledo Program
Program code: 220-38-22-237
NRMP Code: 1579220C0
Program type: University-based
State: Ohio

Address: University of Toledo Medical Center
        3120 Glendale Ave, Toledo, OH 43614-5809
Phone: (419) 383-4590
Fax: (419) 383-3090
Percentage of IMGs in the program: 10%
Minimum USMLE Step 1 Score Requirement: No limits set
Minimum USMLE Step 2 Score Requirement: No limits set
Attempts on any step: Must pass on the first attempt
CS required at time of application: No
USCE Requirement: None
Cut-Off time since graduation: 7 years
Program offers couple match: Yes
Visas Sponsored or accepted: J1 visa

Riverside Methodist Hospitals (OhioHealth) Obstetrics and Gynecology Residency Program

Specialty: Obstetrics and Gynecology OB GYN Residency
Program name: Riverside Methodist Hospitals (OhioHealth) Program
Program code: 220-38-32-235
State: Ohio

Address: Riverside Methodist Hospital
3535 Olentangy River Rd, Columbus, OH 43214
Phone: (614) 566-4882
Fax: (614) 566-1073
Percentage of IMGs in the program: 0%
Minimum USMLE Step 1 Score Requirement: No limits set
Minimum USMLE Step 2 Score Requirement: No limits set
Attempts on any step: No limits set
CS required at time of application: Yes including ECFMG certificate
USCE Requirement: None
Cut-Off time since graduation: No limits set
Program offers couple match: Yes
Visas Sponsored or accepted: J1 visa

Oklahoma

University of Oklahoma Health Sciences Center Obstetrics and Gynecology Residency Program

Specialty: Obstetrics and Gynecology OB GYN Residency

Program name: University of Oklahoma Health Sciences Center Program
Program code: 220-39-11-239
State: Oklahoma
Address: University of Oklahoma Health Sciences Center
920 Stanton L Young Blvd, Oklahoma City, OK 73109
Phone: (405) 271-8470
Fax: (405) 271-8547
Percentage of IMGs in the program: 0%
Minimum USMLE Step 1 Score Requirement: No limits set
Minimum USMLE Step 2 Score Requirement: No limits set
Attempts on any step: Must pass maximum from 3rd attempt
CS required at time of application: No
USCE Requirement: None
Cut-Off time since graduation: No limits set
Program offers couple match: Yes
Visas Sponsored or accepted: J1 visa

University of Oklahoma School of Community Medicine (Tulsa) Obstetrics and Gynecology Residency Program

Specialty: Obstetrics and Gynecology OB GYN Residency

Program name: University of Oklahoma School of Community Medicine (Tulsa) Program
Program code: 220-39-21-240
State: Oklahoma
Address: University of Oklahoma College of Medicine Tulsa
       4502 E 41st St, Tulsa, OK 74135
Phone: (918) 660-8359
Fax: (918) 660-8355
Percentage of IMGs in the program: 10%
Minimum USMLE Step 1 Score Requirement: No limits set
Minimum USMLE Step 2 Score Requirement: No limits set
Attempts on any step: Must pass maximum from the 3rd attempt
CS required at time of application: Yes including ECFMG certificate
USCE Requirement: None
Cut-Off time since graduation: 5 years
Program offers couple match: Yes
Visas Sponsored or accepted: J1 visa and H1b visa

Oregon

Oregon Health & Science University Obstetrics and Gynecology Residency Program

Specialty: Obstetrics and Gynecology OB GYN Residency
Program name: Oregon Health & Science University Program
Program code: 220-40-21-241
Program type: University-based
State: Oregon
Address: Oregon Health & Science University
3181 SW Sam Jackson Park Rd,
Portland, OR 97239
Phone: (503) 494-3106
Fax: (503) 494-5680
Percentage of IMGs in the program: 0%
Minimum USMLE Step 1 Score Requirement: No limits set
Minimum USMLE Step 2 Score Requirement: No limits set
Attempts on any step: Must pass on the first attempt
CS required at time of application: Yes including ECFMG certificate
USCE Requirement: None
Cut-Off time since graduation: No limits set
Program offers couple match: Yes
Visas Sponsored or accepted: J1 visa and H1b visa

Pennsylvania

Lehigh Valley Health Network/University of South Florida College of Medicine Obstetrics and Gynecology Residency Program

Specialty: Obstetrics and Gynecology OB GYN Residency
Program name: Lehigh Valley Health Network/University of South Florida College of Medicine Program
Program code: 220-41-11-243
NRMP Code: 1601220C0
Program type: Community-based university affiliated hospital
State: Pennsylvania
Address: Lehigh Valley Health Network
              707 Hamilton St, Allentown, PA 18105-7017
Phone: (848) 862-3118
Fax: (848) 862-3102
Percentage of IMGs in the program: 10%
Minimum USMLE Step 1 Score Requirement: 210

Minimum USMLE Step 2 Score Requirement:
220
Attempts on any step: No limits set
CS required at time of application: Yes
including ECFMG certificate
USCE Requirement: None
Cut-Off time since graduation: No limits set
Program offers couple match: Yes
Visas Sponsored or accepted: J1 visa and H1b
visa

Main Line Health System/Lankenau Medical Center Obstetrics and Gynecology Residency Program

Specialty: Obstetrics and Gynecology OB
GYN Residency
Program name: Main Line Health
System/Lankenau Medical Center Program
Program code: 220-41-11-249
NRMP Code: 1632220C0
Program type: Community-based
university affiliated hospital
State: Pennsylvania
Address: Lankenau Medical Center
         100 Lancaster Ave, Wynnewood,
PA 19096
Phone: (484) 476-4650
Fax: (484) 476-2422
Percentage of IMGs in the program: 10%

**Minimum USMLE Step 1 Score
Requirement:** No limits set
**Minimum USMLE Step 2 Score
Requirement:** No limits set
Attempts on any step: Must pass on the first attempt
CS required at time of application: Yes including ECFMG certificate
USCE Requirement: Yes
Cut-Off time since graduation: 5 years
Program offers couple match: Yes
Visas Sponsored or accepted: J1 visa and H1b visa

Pennsylvania Hospital of the University of Pennsylvania Health System Obstetrics and Gynecology Residency Program

Specialty: Obstetrics and Gynecology OB GYN Residency
Program name: Pennsylvania Hospital of the University of Pennsylvania Health System Program
Program code: 220-41-11-252
NRMP Code: 1639220C0
Program type: Community-based university affiliated hospital
State: Pennsylvania

Address: Pennsylvania Hospital
800 Spruce St, Philadelphia, PA 19107
Phone: (215) 829-3470
Fax: (215) 829-3973
Percentage of IMGs in the program: 0%
Minimum USMLE Step 1 Score Requirement: No limits set
Minimum USMLE Step 2 Score Requirement: No limits set
Attempts on any step: Must pass on the first attempt
CS required at time of application: Yes including ECFMG certificate
USCE Requirement: None
Cut-Off time since graduation: 5 years
Program offers couple match: Yes
Visas Sponsored or accepted: J1 visa and H1b visa

University of Pennsylvania Obstetrics and Gynecology Residency Program

Specialty: Obstetrics and Gynecology OB GYN Residency
Program name: University of Pennsylvania Program
Program code: 220-41-11-256

Program type: University-based
State: Pennsylvania
Address: Hospital of University of Pennsylvania
3400 Spruce St, Philadelphia, PA
19104-4283
Phone: (215) 662-2459
Fax: (215) 349-5893
Percentage of IMGs in the program: 0%
Minimum USMLE Step 1 Score Requirement:
No limits set
Minimum USMLE Step 2 Score Requirement:
No limits set
Attempts on any step: Must pass on the first
attempt
CS required at time of application: Yes
including ECFMG certificate
USCE Requirement: None
Cut-Off time since graduation: 4 years
Program offers couple match: No
Visas Sponsored or accepted: J1 visa

UPMC Medical Education Obstetrics and Gynecology Residency Program

Specialty: Obstetrics and Gynecology OB GYN
Residency
Program name: UPMC Medical Education
Program
Program code: 220-41-11-258
NRMP Code: 1652220C0

Program type: University-based
State: Pennsylvania
Address: Magee-Womens Hospital
          300 Halket St, Pittsburgh, PA 15213-3180
Phone: (412) 641-1092
Fax: (412) 641-2649
Percentage of IMGs in the program: 0%
Minimum USMLE Step 1 Score Requirement: No limits set
Minimum USMLE Step 2 Score Requirement: No limits set
Attempts on any step: Must pass on the first attempt
CS required at time of application: Yes including ECFMG certificate
USCE Requirement: 12 months
Cut-Off time since graduation: No limits set
Program offers couple match: Yes
Visas Sponsored or accepted: J1 visa

Allegheny Health Network Medical Education Consortium (WPH) Obstetrics and Gynecology Residency Program

Specialty: Obstetrics and Gynecology OB GYN Residency
Program name: Allegheny Health Network Medical Education Consortium (WPH) Program

Program code: 220-41-11-261
NRMP Code: 1659220C0
Program type: Community-based university affiliated hospital
State: Pennsylvania
Address: Western Pennsylvania Hospital
4800 Friendship Ave, Pittsburgh, PA 15224
Phone: (412) 578-5587
Fax: (412) 578-4477
Percentage of IMGs in the program: 15%
Minimum USMLE Step 1 Score Requirement: 210
Minimum USMLE Step 2 Score Requirement: 210
Attempts on any step: No limits set
CS required at time of application: Yes including ECFMG certificate
USCE Requirement: None
Cut-Off time since graduation: No limits set
Program offers couple match: Yes
Visas Sponsored or accepted: J1 visa

York Hospital Obstetrics and Gynecology Residency Program

Specialty: Obstetrics and Gynecology OB GYN Residency
Program name: York Hospital Program
Program code: 220-41-11-263

NRMP Code: 1674220C0
Program type: Community-based university affiliated hospital
State: Pennsylvania
Address: York Hospital
        1001 S George St, York, PA 17405
Phone: (717) 851-2348
Fax: (717) 851-2426
Percentage of IMGs in the program: 0%
Minimum USMLE Step 1 Score Requirement: No limits set
Minimum USMLE Step 2 Score Requirement: No limits set
Attempts on any step: No limits set
CS required at time of application: No
USCE Requirement: None
Cut-Off time since graduation: No limits set
Program offers couple match: No
Visas Sponsored or accepted: J1 visa and H1b visa

Abington Memorial Hospital Obstetrics and Gynecology Residency Program

Specialty: Obstetrics and Gynecology OB GYN Residency
Program name: Abington Memorial Hospital Program
Program code: 220-41-12-242

NRMP Code: 1600220C0
Program type: Community-based university affiliated hospital
State: Pennsylvania
Address: Abington Memorial Hospital
1200 Old York Rd, Abington, PA 19001
Phone: (215) 481-4231
Fax: (215) 481-2048
Percentage of IMGs in the program: 0%
Minimum USMLE Step 1 Score Requirement: No limits set
Minimum USMLE Step 2 Score Requirement: No limits set
Attempts on any step: No limits set
CS required at time of application: Yes including ECFMG certificate
USCE Requirement: None
Cut-Off time since graduation: No limits set
Program offers couple match: Yes
Visas Sponsored or accepted: J1 visa and H1b visa

Geisinger Health System Obstetrics and Gynecology Residency Program

Specialty: Obstetrics and Gynecology OB GYN Residency
Program name: Geisinger Health System Program
Program code: 220-41-12-245

State: Pennsylvania
Address: Geisinger Medical Center
100 N Academy Ave, Danville, PA 17822-2920
Phone: (570) 271-5936
Fax: (570) 271-5819
Percentage of IMGs in the program: 15%
Minimum USMLE Step 1 Score Requirement: No limits set
Minimum USMLE Step 2 Score Requirement: No limits set
Attempts on any step: Must pass on the first attempt
CS required at time of application: Yes including ECFMG certificate
USCE Requirement: None
Cut-Off time since graduation: 5 years
Program offers couple match: Yes
Visas Sponsored or accepted: J1 visa

Reading Hospital Obstetrics and Gynecology Residency Program

Specialty: Obstetrics and Gynecology OB GYN Residency
Program name: Reading Hospital Program
Program code: 220-41-12-262
NRMP Code: 1661220C0
Program type: Community-based university affiliated hospital

State: Pennsylvania
Address: Reading Hospital
          Sixth Ave & Spruce Sts, Reading, PA 19612
Phone: (484) 628-8614
Fax: (484) 628-9292
Percentage of IMGs in the program: 0%
Minimum USMLE Step 1 Score Requirement: No limits set
Minimum USMLE Step 2 Score Requirement: No limits set
Attempts on any step: No limits set
CS required at time of application: Yes including ECFMG certificate
USCE Requirement: None
Cut-Off time since graduation: No limits set
Program offers couple match: Yes
Visas Sponsored or accepted: J1 visa and H1b visa

Penn State Milton S Hershey Medical Center Obstetrics and Gynecology Residency Program

Specialty: Obstetrics and Gynecology OB GYN Residency
Program name: Penn State Milton S Hershey Medical Center Program
Program code: 220-41-21-246
NRMP Code: 1617220C0

Program type: University-based
State: Pennsylvania
Address: Penn State Hershey Medical Center
500 University Dr, Hershey, PA 17033-0850
Phone: (717) 531-5394
Fax: (717) 531-0066
Percentage of IMGs in the program: 5%
Minimum USMLE Step 1 Score Requirement:
No limits set
Minimum USMLE Step 2 Score Requirement:
No limits set
Attempts on any step: No limits set
CS required at time of application: No
USCE Requirement: None
Cut-Off time since graduation: No limits set
Program offers couple match: Yes
Visas Sponsored or accepted: J1 visa

Albert Einstein Healthcare Network Obstetrics and Gynecology Residency Program

Specialty: Obstetrics and Gynecology OB GYN
Residency
Program name: Albert Einstein Healthcare
Network Program
Program code: 220-41-21-247
NRMP Code: 1631220C0
Program type: Community-based

State: Pennsylvania
Address: Albert Einstein Medical Center
          5501 Old York Rd, Philadelphia, PA
19141-3098
Phone: (215) 456-8261
Fax: (215) 456-4958
Percentage of IMGs in the program: 50%
Minimum USMLE Step 1 Score Requirement:
220
Minimum USMLE Step 2 Score Requirement:
220
Attempts on any step: No limits set
CS required at time of application: Yes
including ECFMG certificate
USCE Requirement: None
Cut-Off time since graduation: No limits set
Program offers couple match: Yes
Visas Sponsored or accepted: J1 visa and H1b
visa

Drexel University College of Medicine/Hahnemann University Hospital Obstetrics and Gynecology Residency Program

Specialty: Obstetrics and Gynecology OB GYN
Residency
Program name: Drexel University College of
Medicine/Hahnemann University Hospital
Program

Program code: 220-41-21-250
NRMP Code: 1849220C0
Program type: University-based
State: Pennsylvania
Address: Drexel University College of Medicine
          245 N 15th St, Philadelphia, PA
19102-1192
Phone: (215) 762-8220
Fax: (215) 762-1470
Percentage of IMGs in the program: 40%
Minimum USMLE Step 1 Score Requirement:
No limits set
Minimum USMLE Step 2 Score Requirement:
No limits set
Attempts on any step: No limits set
CS required at time of application: Yes
including ECFMG certificate
USCE Requirement: None
Cut-Off time since graduation: 4 years
Program offers couple match: Yes
Visas Sponsored or accepted: J1 visa

Temple University Hospital Obstetrics and Gynecology Residency Program

Specialty: Obstetrics and Gynecology OB GYN
Residency
Program name: Temple University Hospital
Program

Program code: 220-41-21-254
State: Pennsylvania
Address: Temple University Hospital
         3401 N Broad St, Philadelphia, PA 19140
Phone: (215) 707-3187
Fax: (215) 707-1387
Percentage of IMGs in the program: 0% (Occasionally 1 match)
Minimum USMLE Step 1 Score Requirement: No limits set
Minimum USMLE Step 2 Score Requirement: No limits set
Attempts on any step: No limits set
CS required at time of application: Yes including ECFMG certificate
USCE Requirement: None
Cut-Off time since graduation: 5 years
Program offers couple match: No
Visas Sponsored or accepted: J1 visa and H1b visa

Thomas Jefferson University Obstetrics and Gynecology Residency Program

Specialty: Obstetrics and Gynecology OB GYN Residency
Program name: Thomas Jefferson University Program

Program code: 220-41-21-255
NRMP Code: 1630220C0
Program type: University-based
State: Pennsylvania
Address: Thomas Jefferson University Hospital
833 Chestnut St, Philadelphia, PA 19107
Phone: (215) 955-1085
Fax: (215) 955-5041
Percentage of IMGs in the program: 0%
Minimum USMLE Step 1 Score Requirement: No limits set
Minimum USMLE Step 2 Score Requirement: No limits set
Attempts on any step: Must pass on the first attempt
CS required at time of application: No
USCE Requirement: None
Cut-Off time since graduation: 5 years
Program offers couple match: Yes
Visas Sponsored or accepted: J1 visa and H1b visa

Crozer-Chester Medical Center Obstetrics and Gynecology Residency Program

Specialty: Obstetrics and Gynecology OB GYN Residency

Program name: Crozer-Chester Medical Center Program
Program code: 220-41-21-367
NRMP Code: 3185220C0
Program type: Community-based university affiliated hospital
State: Pennsylvania
Address: Crozer-Chester Medical Center
One Medical Center Blvd, Upland, PA 19013
Phone: (610) 447-7612
Fax: (610) 447-7615
Percentage of IMGs in the program: 60%
Minimum USMLE Step 1 Score Requirement: No limits set
Minimum USMLE Step 2 Score Requirement: No limits set
Attempts on any step: No limits set
CS required at time of application: No
USCE Requirement: None
Cut-Off time since graduation: No limits set
Program offers couple match: No
Visas Sponsored or accepted: J1 visa and H1b visa

St Luke's Hospital Obstetrics and Gynecology Residency Program

Specialty: Obstetrics and Gynecology OB GYN Residency

Program name: St Luke's Hospital Program
Program code: 220-41-31-244
NRMP Code: 1605220C0
Program type: Community-based university affiliated hospital
State: Pennsylvania
Address: St Luke's University Health Network
             801 Ostrum St, Bethlehem, PA 18015
Phone: (484) 526-4670
Fax: (484) 526-2381
Percentage of IMGs in the program: 40%
Minimum USMLE Step 1 Score Requirement: 220
Minimum USMLE Step 2 Score Requirement: 220
Attempts on any step: No limits set
CS required at time of application: No
USCE Requirement: None
Cut-Off time since graduation: No limits set
Program offers couple match: No
Visas Sponsored or accepted: J1 visa and H1b visa

Rhode Island

Brown University (Women and Infants Hospital of Rhode Island) Obstetrics and Gynecology Residency Program

Specialty: Obstetrics and Gynecology OB GYN Residency
Program name: Brown University (Women and Infants Hospital of Rhode Island) Program
Program code: 220-43-21-269
NRMP Code: 2793220C0
Program type: University-based
State: Rhode Island
Address: Women and Infants Hospital Rhode Island

      101 Dudley St, Providence, RI 02905
Phone: (401) 274-1122   Ext: 41845
Fax: (401) 453-7696
Percentage of IMGs in the program: 0%
Minimum USMLE Step 1 Score Requirement: No limits set
Minimum USMLE Step 2 Score Requirement: No limits set
Attempts on any step: No limits set
CS required at time of application: Yes including ECFMG certificate
USCE Requirement: None
Cut-Off time since graduation: 5 years
Program offers couple match: Yes
Visas Sponsored or accepted: J1 visa

South Carolina

Greenville Health System/University of South Carolina Obstetrics and Gynecology Residency Program

Specialty: Obstetrics and Gynecology
Program name: Greenville Health System/University of South Carolina Program
Program code: 220-45-11-272
NRMP Code: 1683220C0
Program type: University-based
State: South Carolina
Address: Greenville Health System, Suite 470, 890 W Faris Rd, Greenville, SC 29605-4253
Phone: (864) 455-7887
Fax: (864) 455-6875
Percentage of IMGs in the program: 0%
Minimum USMLE Step 1 Score Requirement: No limits set
Minimum USMLE Step 2 Score Requirement: No limits set
Attempts on any step: No limits set

CS required at time of application: Yes including ECFMG certificate
USCE Requirement: None
Cut-Off time since graduation: No limits set
Program offers couple match: Yes
Visas Sponsored or accepted: J1 visa

Palmetto Health/University of South Carolina School of Medicine Obstetrics and Gynecology Residency Program

Specialty: Obstetrics and Gynecology
Program name: Palmetto Health/University of South Carolina School of Medicine Program
Program code: 220-45-11-271
State: South Carolina
Address: Palmetto Health Richland Hospital, Suite 208,
         Two Medical Park, Columbia, SC 29203
Phone: (803) 545-5702
Fax: (803) 434-4699
Percentage of IMGs in the program: 10%
Minimum USMLE Step 1 Score Requirement: No limits set
Minimum USMLE Step 2 Score Requirement: No limits set
Attempts on any step: No limits set

CS required at time of application: Yes including ECFMG certificate
USCE Requirement: None
Cut-Off time since graduation: 5 years
Program offers couple match: Yes
Visas Sponsored or accepted: No visa

Medical University of South Carolina Obstetrics and Gynecology Residency Program

Specialty: Obstetrics and Gynecology
Program name: Medical University of South Carolina Program
Program code: 220-45-21-270
NRMP Code: 1680220C0
Program type: University-based
State: South Carolina
Address: Medical University of South Carolina, Suite 634 PO Box 250619,
          96 Jonathan Lucas St, Charleston, SC 29425-2233
Phone: (843) 792-7108
Fax: (843) 792-0533
Percentage of IMGs in the program: 0%
Minimum USMLE Step 1 Score Requirement: No limits set
Minimum USMLE Step 2 Score Requirement: No limits set

Attempts on any step: Must pass on first attempt
CS required at time of application: No
USCE Requirement: Yes
Cut-Off time since graduation: 2 years
Program offers couple match: Yes
Visas Sponsored or accepted: J1 visa

Tennessee

University of Tennessee College of Medicine Obstetrics and Gynecology Residency Program

Specialty: Obstetrics and Gynecology OB GYN Residency
Program name: University of Tennessee College of Medicine Program
Program code: 220-47-00-362
Program type: University-based
State: Tennessee
Address: St Thomas Midtown Hospital
              2000 Church St, Nashville, TN 37236
Phone: (615) 222-4059
Fax: (615) 222-6464
Percentage of IMGs in the program: 0%
Minimum USMLE Step 1 Score Requirement: 220

Minimum USMLE Step 2 Score Requirement:
220
Attempts on any step: Must pass on the first attempt
CS required at time of application: Yes including ECFMG certificate
USCE Requirement: 1 month
Cut-Off time since graduation: 5 years
Program offers couple match: Yes
Visas Sponsored or accepted: J1 visa

University of Tennessee Medical Center at Knoxville Obstetrics and Gynecology Residency Program

Specialty: Obstetrics and Gynecology OB GYN Residency
Program name: University of Tennessee Medical Center at Knoxville Program
Program code: 220-47-11-275
NRMP Code: 1839220C0
Program type: Community-based university affiliated hospital
State: Tennessee
Address: University of Tennessee Memorial Hospital
        1924 Alcoa Hwy, Knoxville, TN 37920
Phone: (865) 305-9584
Fax: (865) 305-6822
Percentage of IMGs in the program: 0%

Minimum USMLE Step 1 Score Requirement: No limits set
Minimum USMLE Step 2 Score Requirement: No limits set
Attempts on any step: No limits set
CS required at time of application: Yes including ECFMG certificate
USCE Requirement: None
Cut-Off time since graduation: No limits set
Program offers couple match: Yes
Visas Sponsored or accepted: J1 visa

University of Tennessee College of Medicine at Chattanooga Obstetrics and Gynecology Residency Program

Specialty: Obstetrics and Gynecology OB GYN Residency
Program name: University of Tennessee College of Medicine at Chattanooga Program
Program code: 220-47-21-274
NRMP Code: 1689220C0
Program type: University-based
State: Tennessee
Address: University of Tennessee College of Medicine-Chattanooga
          979 E Third St, Chattanooga, TN 37403
Phone: (423) 778-7515
Fax: (423) 778-7522

Percentage of IMGs in the program: 20%
Minimum USMLE Step 1 Score Requirement: No limits set
Minimum USMLE Step 2 Score Requirement: No limits set
Attempts on any step: Must pass on the first attempt
CS required at time of application: Yes including ECFMG certificate
USCE Requirement: None
Cut-Off time since graduation: No limits set
Program offers couple match: Yes
Visas Sponsored or accepted: J1 visa

University of Tennessee Obstetrics and Gynecology Residency Program

Specialty: Obstetrics and Gynecology OB GYN Residency
Program name: University of Tennessee Program
Program code: 220-47-21-276
NRMP Code: 1844220C0
Program type: University-based
State: Tennessee
Address: University of Tennessee Health Science Center
853 Jefferson Ave, Memphis, TN 38163
Phone: (901) 448-4795

Fax: (901) 448-7075
Percentage of IMGs in the program: 15%
Minimum USMLE Step 1 Score Requirement: No limits set
Minimum USMLE Step 2 Score Requirement: No limits set
Attempts on any step: No limits set
CS required at time of application: No
USCE Requirement: None
Cut-Off time since graduation: 5 years unless clinically active for at least 2 years during the last 7 years
Program offers couple match: Yes
Visas Sponsored or accepted: J1 visa

Vanderbilt University Obstetrics and Gynecology Residency Program

Specialty: Obstetrics and Gynecology OB GYN Residency
Program name: Vanderbilt University Program
Program code: 220-47-21-278
NRMP Code: 1702220C0
Program type: University-based
State: Tennessee
Address: Vanderbilt University Medical Center
1611 21st Ave S, Nashville, TN 37232-2521
Phone: (615) 343-8801
Fax: (615) 343-8806

Percentage of IMGs in the program: 10%
Minimum USMLE Step 1 Score Requirement: 215
Minimum USMLE Step 2 Score Requirement: 215
Attempts on any step: No limits set
CS required at time of application: Yes including ECFMG certificate
USCE Requirement: Yes
Cut-Off time since graduation: 5 years
Program offers couple match: Yes
Visas Sponsored or accepted: J1 visa

East Tennessee State University Obstetrics and Gynecology Residency Program

Specialty: Obstetrics and Gynecology OB GYN Residency
Program name: East Tennessee State University Program
Program code: 220-47-21-341
NRMP Code: 2066220C0
Program type: University-based
State: Tennessee
Address: ETSU James H Quillen College of Medicine
PO Box 70569, Johnson City, TN 37614
Phone: (423) 439-6262

Fax: (423) 439-6766
Percentage of IMGs in the program: 15%
Minimum USMLE Step 1 Score Requirement: 220
Minimum USMLE Step 2 Score Requirement: 220
Attempts on any step: Must pass maximum on the 2nd attempt
CS required at time of application: Yes including ECFMG certificate
USCE Requirement: 12 months
Cut-Off time since graduation: 3 years
Program offers couple match: Yes
Visas Sponsored or accepted: J1 visa

Meharry Medical College Obstetrics and Gynecology Residency Program

Specialty: Obstetrics and Gynecology OB GYN Residency
Program name: Meharry Medical College Program
Program code: 220-47-23-361
State: Tennessee
Address: Meharry Medical College
          1005 Dr D B Todd Jr Blvd, Nashville, TN 37208
Phone: (615) 327-5547
Fax: (615) 327-6296
Percentage of IMGs in the program: 0%

Minimum USMLE Step 1 Score Requirement: No limits set

Minimum USMLE Step 2 Score Requirement: No limits set

Attempts on any step: No limits set

CS required at time of application: Yes including ECFMG certificate

USCE Requirement: None

Cut-Off time since graduation: 5 years unless in research or clinically active

Program offers couple match: Yes

Visas Sponsored or accepted: No visa

Texas

University of Texas RGV (DHR) Obstetrics and Gynecology Residency Program

Specialty: Obstetrics and Gynecology OB GYN Residency

Program name: University of Texas RGV (DHR) Program

Program code: 220-48-00-361

State: Texas

Address: University of Texas Rio Grande Valley - Doctors Hospital at Renaissance
2821 Michaelangelo Dr, Edinburg, TX 78539
Phone: (956) 362-3594
Fax: (956) 362-3598
Percentage of IMGs in the program: 10%
Minimum USMLE Step 1 Score Requirement: No limits set
Minimum USMLE Step 2 Score Requirement: No limits set
Attempts on any step: No limits set
CS required at time of application: Yes including ECFMG certificate
USCE Requirement: None
Cut-Off time since graduation: No limits set
Program offers couple match: Yes
Visas Sponsored or accepted: J1 visa

Texas Tech University Health Sciences Center Paul L Foster School of Medicine Obstetrics and Gynecology Residency Program

Specialty: Obstetrics and Gynecology OB GYN Residency
Program name: Texas Tech University Health Sciences Center Paul L Foster School of Medicine Program
Program code: 220-48-11-315

NRMP Code: 1710220C0
Program type: University-based
State: Texas
Address: Texas Tech University HSC Paul L
Foster School of Medicine
        4800 Alberta Ave, El Paso, TX 79905
Phone: (915) 215-5020
Fax: (915) 545-0901
Percentage of IMGs in the program: 5%
Minimum USMLE Step 1 Score Requirement:
210
Minimum USMLE Step 2 Score Requirement:
210
Attempts on any step: Must pass on the first
attempt
CS required at time of application: Yes
including ECFMG certificate
USCE Requirement: None
Cut-Off time since graduation: No limits set
Program offers couple match: Yes
Visas Sponsored or accepted: No visa

University of Texas at Austin Dell Medical School Obstetrics and Gynecology Residency Program

Specialty: Obstetrics and Gynecology OB GYN
Residency
Program name: University of Texas at Austin
Dell Medical School Program

Program code: 220-48-12-360
NRMP Code: 2835220C2
Program type: Community-based university affiliated hospital
State: Texas
Address: University of Texas at Austin Dell Medical School
1313 Red River St, Austin, TX 78701
Phone: (512) 324-7036
Fax: (512) 324-7971
Percentage of IMGs in the program: 0%
Minimum USMLE Step 1 Score Requirement: 210
Minimum USMLE Step 2 Score Requirement: 210
Attempts on any step: Must pass on the first attempt
CS required at time of application: No
USCE Requirement: None
Cut-Off time since graduation: 4 years
Program offers couple match: Yes
Visas Sponsored or accepted: J1 visa

University of Texas Medical Branch Hospitals Obstetrics and Gynecology Residency Program

Specialty: Obstetrics and Gynecology OB GYN Residency

Program name: University of Texas Medical Branch Hospitals Program
Program code: 220-48-21-285
NRMP Code: 1714220C0
Program type: University-based
State: Texas
Address: University of Texas Med Branch Hospitals

   301 University Blvd, Galveston, TX 77555-0587
Phone: (409) 772-2999
Fax: (409) 772-5803
Percentage of IMGs in the program: 10%
Minimum USMLE Step 1 Score Requirement: No limits set
Minimum USMLE Step 2 Score Requirement: No limits set
Attempts on any step: Must pass maximum from the 3rd attempt
CS required at time of application: No
USCE Requirement: 12 months
Cut-Off time since graduation: 3 years
Program offers couple match: Yes
Visas Sponsored or accepted: J1 visa

University of Texas Health Science Center at Houston (Memorial Hermann Hospital) Obstetrics and Gynecology Residency Program

Specialty: Obstetrics and Gynecology OB GYN Residency
Program name: University of Texas Health Science Center at Houston (Memorial Hermann Hospital) Program
Program code: 220-48-21-289
NRMP Code: 2923220C0
Program type: University-based
State: Texas
Address: University of Texas Medical School Houston
6431 Fannin St, Houston, TX 77030
Phone: (713) 500-6397
Fax: (713) 500-0798
Percentage of IMGs in the program: 10%
Minimum USMLE Step 1 Score Requirement: No limits set
Minimum USMLE Step 2 Score Requirement: No limits set
Attempts on any step: Must pass maximum on the 3rd attempt
CS required at time of application: Yes including ECFMG certificate
USCE Requirement: None
Cut-Off time since graduation: No limits set
Program offers couple match: Yes
Visas Sponsored or accepted: J1 visa

Texas Tech University (Lubbock) Obstetrics and Gynecology Residency Program

Specialty: Obstetrics and Gynecology OB GYN Residency
Program name: Texas Tech University (Lubbock) Program
Program code: 220-48-21-290
NRMP Code: 2973220C0
Program type: Community-based university affiliated hospital
State: Texas
Address: Texas Tech University HSC Lubbock
3601 4th St, Lubbock, TX 79430
Phone: (806) 743-3039
Fax: (806) 743-2174
Percentage of IMGs in the program: 40%
Minimum USMLE Step 1 Score Requirement: No limits set
Minimum USMLE Step 2 Score Requirement: No limits set
Attempts on any step: Must pass maximum on the 3rd attempt
CS required at time of application: Yes including ECFMG certificate
USCE Requirement: None
Cut-Off time since graduation: No limits set
Program offers couple match: Yes
Visas Sponsored or accepted: J1 visa

University of Texas Health Science Center School of Medicine at San Antonio Obstetrics and Gynecology Residency Program

Specialty: Obstetrics and Gynecology OB GYN Residency
Program name: University of Texas Health Science Center School of Medicine at San Antonio Program
Program code: 220-48-21-292
NRMP Code: 1722220C0
Program type: University-based
State: Texas
Address: University of Texas HSC San Antonio 7703 Floyd Curl Dr, San Antonio, TX 78229-3900
Phone: (210) 567-4953
Fax: (210) 567-3485
Percentage of IMGs in the program: 0%
Minimum USMLE Step 1 Score Requirement: No limits set
Minimum USMLE Step 2 Score Requirement: No limits set
Attempts on any step: No limits set
CS required at time of application: Yes including ECFMG certificate
USCE Requirement: None
Cut-Off time since graduation: No limits set
Program offers couple match: Yes

Visas Sponsored or accepted: J1 visa

Texas A&M College of Medicine-Scott and White Obstetrics and Gynecology Residency Program

Specialty: Obstetrics and Gynecology OB GYN Residency
Program name: Texas A&M College of Medicine-Scott and White Program
Program code: 220-48-21-293
NRMP Code: 1725220C0
Program type: University-based
State: Texas
Address: Scott and White Memorial Hospital
                  2401 S 31st St, Temple, TX 76508-0001
Phone: (254) 724-7588
Fax: (254) 724-7976
Percentage of IMGs in the program: 0%
Minimum USMLE Step 1 Score Requirement: No limits set
Minimum USMLE Step 2 Score Requirement: No limits set
Attempts on any step: Must pass maximum on the 3rd attempt
CS required at time of application: Yes including ECFMG certificate
USCE Requirement: None
Cut-Off time since graduation: No limits set

Program offers couple match: Yes
Visas Sponsored or accepted: J1 visa

Texas Tech University (Amarillo) Obstetrics and Gynecology Residency Program

Specialty: Obstetrics and Gynecology OB GYN Residency
Program name: Texas Tech University (Amarillo) Program
Program code: 220-48-21-320
NRMP Code: 2993220C0
Program type: University-based
State: Texas
Address: Texas Tech University HSC Amarillo
1400 Coulter Rd, Amarillo, TX 79106
Phone: (806) 414-9006
Fax: (806) 354-5516
Percentage of IMGs in the program: 0%
Minimum USMLE Step 1 Score Requirement: No limits set
Minimum USMLE Step 2 Score Requirement: No limits set
Attempts on any step: Must pass maximum on the 3rd attempt
CS required at time of application: No
USCE Requirement: None
Cut-Off time since graduation: No limits set
Program offers couple match: Yes

Visas Sponsored or accepted: J1 visa

Texas Tech University (Permian Basin) Obstetrics and Gynecology Residency Program

Specialty: Obstetrics and Gynecology OB GYN Residency
Program name: Texas Tech University (Permian Basin) Program
Program code: 220-48-21-331
NRMP Code: 3124220C0
Program type: University-based
State: Texas
Address: Texas Tech University HSC Odessa
701 W 5th St, Odessa, TX 79763-4362
Phone: (432) 703-5050
Fax: (432) 335-5240
Percentage of IMGs in the program: 10%
Minimum USMLE Step 1 Score Requirement: No limits set
Minimum USMLE Step 2 Score Requirement: No limits set
Attempts on any step: Must pass maximum on the 3rd attempt
CS required at time of application: Yes including ECFMG certificate
USCE Requirement: Yes
Cut-Off time since graduation: No limits set
Program offers couple match: Yes

Visas Sponsored or accepted: J1 visa

University of Texas Health Science Center at Houston (Lyndon B Johnson General Hospital) Obstetrics and Gynecology Residency Program

Specialty: Obstetrics and Gynecology OB GYN Residency
Program name: University of Texas Health Science Center at Houston (Lyndon B Johnson General Hospital) Program
Program code: 220-48-21-334
NRMP Code: 2923220C1
Program type: University-based
State: Texas
Address: Lyndon B Johnson General Hospital
5656 Kelley St, Houston, TX 77026
Phone: (713) 566-5735
Fax: (713) 566-4521
Percentage of IMGs in the program: 15%
Minimum USMLE Step 1 Score Requirement: No limits set
Minimum USMLE Step 2 Score Requirement: No limits set
Attempts on any step: Must pass maximum on the 3rd attempt

CS required at time of application: Yes including ECFMG certificate
USCE Requirement: None
Cut-Off time since graduation: No limits set
Program offers couple match: Yes
Visas Sponsored or accepted: J1 visa

John Peter Smith Hospital (Tarrant County Hospital District) Obstetrics and Gynecology Residency Program

Specialty: Obstetrics and Gynecology OB GYN Residency
Program name: John Peter Smith Hospital (Tarrant County Hospital District) Program
Program code: 220-48-22-284
NRMP Code: 1711220C0
Program type: Community-based
State: Texas
Address: John Peter Smith Hospital
            1500 S Main St, Fort Worth, TX 76104
Phone: (817) 927-1142
Fax: (817) 927-1162
Percentage of IMGs in the program: 0%
Minimum USMLE Step 1 Score Requirement: No limits set
Minimum USMLE Step 2 Score Requirement: No limits set
Attempts on any step: Must pass on the first attempt

CS required at time of application: No
USCE Requirement: None
Cut-Off time since graduation: No limits set
Program offers couple match: Yes
Visas Sponsored or accepted: No visa

Baylor University Medical Center Obstetrics and Gynecology Residency Program

Specialty: Obstetrics and Gynecology OB GYN Residency
Program name: Baylor University Medical Center Program
Program code: 220-48-31-280
NRMP Code: 1706220C0
State: Texas
Address: Baylor University Medical Center
3500 Gaston Ave, Dallas, TX 75246
Phone: (214) 820-6378
Fax: (214) 820-6880
Percentage of IMGs in the program: 0%
Minimum USMLE Step 1 Score Requirement: 210
Minimum USMLE Step 2 Score Requirement: 210
Attempts on any step: Must pass on the first attempt
CS required at time of application: Yes including ECFMG certificate

USCE Requirement: None
Cut-Off time since graduation: 6 years
Program offers couple match: Yes
Visas Sponsored or accepted: J1 visa

Methodist Health System Dallas Obstetrics and Gynecology Residency Program

Specialty: Obstetrics and Gynecology OB GYN Residency
Program name: Methodist Health System Dallas Program
Program code: 220-48-31-281
NRMP Code: 1707220C0
Program type: Community-based
State: Texas
Address: Methodist Health System Dallas
1441 N Beckley Ave, Dallas, TX 75203
Phone: (214) 947-2331
Fax: (214) 947-2361
Percentage of IMGs in the program: 10%
Minimum USMLE Step 1 Score Requirement: 210
Minimum USMLE Step 2 Score Requirement: 210
Attempts on any step: Must pass on the first attempt
CS required at time of application: Yes including ECFMG certificate

USCE Requirement: None
Cut-Off time since graduation: 2 years
Program offers couple match: Yes
Visas Sponsored or accepted: No visa

University of Texas Southwestern Medical School Obstetrics and Gynecology Residency Program

Specialty: Obstetrics and Gynecology OB GYN Residency
Program name: University of Texas Southwestern Medical School Program
Program code: 220-48-31-282
NRMP Code: 2835220C0
Program type: University-based
State: Texas
Address: University of Texas Southwestern Medical Center
        5323 Harry Hines Blvd, Dallas, TX 75390-9032
Phone: (214) 648-2986
Fax: (214) 648-4566
Percentage of IMGs in the program: 0%
Minimum USMLE Step 1 Score Requirement: No limits set
Minimum USMLE Step 2 Score Requirement: No limits set
Attempts on any step: No limits set
CS required at time of application: No

USCE Requirement: None
Cut-Off time since graduation: No limits set
Program offers couple match: Yes
Visas Sponsored or accepted: J1 visa

Baylor College of Medicine Obstetrics and Gynecology Residency Program

Specialty: Obstetrics and Gynecology OB GYN Residency
Program name: Baylor College of Medicine Program
Program code: 220-48-31-286
NRMP Code: 1716220C0
State: Texas
Address: Baylor College of Medicine
One Baylor Plaza, Houston, TX 77030
Phone: (832) 826-7372
Fax: (832) 825-9352
Percentage of IMGs in the program: 0%
Minimum USMLE Step 1 Score Requirement: 230
Minimum USMLE Step 2 Score Requirement: 230
Attempts on any step: Must pass on the first attempt
CS required at time of application: Yes including ECFMG certificate
USCE Requirement: None

Cut-Off time since graduation: 3 years
Program offers couple match: Yes
Visas Sponsored or accepted: J1 visa

Methodist Hospital (Houston) Obstetrics and Gynecology Residency Program

Specialty: Obstetrics and Gynecology OB GYN Residency
Program name: Methodist Hospital (Houston) Program
Program code: 220-48-31-288
NRMP Code: 1167220C0
Program type: Community-based
State: Texas
Address: Houston Methodist Hospital
1401 St Joseph Pkwy, Houston, TX 77002
Phone: (713) 756-8374
Fax: (713) 657-7191
Percentage of IMGs in the program: 5%
Minimum USMLE Step 1 Score Requirement: 220
Minimum USMLE Step 2 Score Requirement: 230
Attempts on any step: Must pass maximum from the 2nd attempt
CS required at time of application: No
USCE Requirement: None

Cut-Off time since graduation: 3 years
Program offers couple match: Yes
Visas Sponsored or accepted: J1 visa and H1b visa

Utah

University of Utah Obstetrics and Gynecology Residency Program

Specialty: Obstetrics and Gynecology
Program name: University of Utah Program
Program code: 220-49-21-294
NRMP Code: 1732220C0
Program type: University-based
State: Utah
Address: University of Utah Medical Center
　　　　　30 N 1900 E, Salt Lake City, UT 84132
Phone: (801) 581-5501
Fax: (801) 585-5146
Percentage of IMGs in the program: 0%
Minimum USMLE Step 1 Score Requirement: No limits set
Minimum USMLE Step 2 Score Requirement: No limits set
Attempts on any step: No limits set

CS required at time of application: Yes
including ECFMG certificate and Step 3
USCE Requirement: Yes
Cut-Off time since graduation: No limits set
Program offers couple match: Yes
Visas Sponsored or accepted: J1 visa

Vermont

University of Vermont/Fletcher Allen Health Care Obstetrics and Gynecology Residency Program

Specialty: Obstetrics and Gynecology
Program name: University of Vermont/Fletcher Allen Health Care Program
Program code: 220-50-21-295
NRMP Code:
Program type:
State: Vermont
Address: University of Vermont FAHC
          111 Colchester Ave, Burlington, VT 05401
Phone: (802) 847-4736

Fax: (802) 847-5626
Percentage of IMGs in the program: 0%
Minimum USMLE Step 1 Score Requirement: No limits set
Minimum USMLE Step 2 Score Requirement: No limits set
Attempts on any step: No limits set
CS required at time of application: Yes including ECFMG certificate
USCE Requirement: Yes within the last 2 years
Cut-Off time since graduation: 2 years
Program offers couple match: Yes
Visas Sponsored or accepted: J1 visa

Virginia

Inova Fairfax Medical Campus Obstetrics and Gynecology Residency Program

Specialty: Obstetrics and Gynecology
Program name: Inova Fairfax Medical Campus Program
Program code: 220-51-00-301
State: Virginia
Address: Women's & Children's Hospital
          3300 Gallows Rd, Falls Church, VA 22042

Phone: (703) 776-2745
Fax: (866) 291-4915
Percentage of IMGs in the program: 40%
Minimum USMLE Step 1 Score Requirement:
No limits set
Minimum USMLE Step 2 Score Requirement:
No limits set
Attempts on any step: Must pass on first
attempt
CS required at time of application: Yes
USCE Requirement: None
Cut-Off time since graduation: 5 years
preferred
Program offers couple match: Yes
Visas Sponsored or accepted: J1 visa and H1b
visa

University of Virginia Obstetrics and Gynecology Residency Program

Specialty: Obstetrics and Gynecology
Program name: University of Virginia Program
Program code: 220-51-11-296
NRMP Code: 1737220C0
Program type: University-based
State: Virginia
Address: University of Virginia Health System
         PO Box 800712, Charlottesville, VA
22908

Phone: (434) 924-9930
Fax: (434) 243-3442
Percentage of IMGs in the program: 0%
Minimum USMLE Step 1 Score Requirement: 210
Minimum USMLE Step 2 Score Requirement: 210
Attempts on any step: Must pass on first attempt
CS required at time of application: Yes including ECFMG certificate
USCE Requirement: None
Cut-Off time since graduation: No limits set
Program offers couple match: Yes
Visas Sponsored or accepted: J1 visa

Riverside Regional Medical Center Obstetrics and Gynecology Residency Program

Specialty: Obstetrics and Gynecology
Program name: Riverside Regional Medical Center Program
Program code: 220-51-11-297
NRMP Code: 1739220C0
Program type: Community-based
State: Virginia
Address: Riverside Regional Medical Center
          500 J Clyde Morris Blvd, Newport News, VA 23601

Phone: (757) 594-4737
Fax: (757) 594-3184
Percentage of IMGs in the program: 40%
Minimum USMLE Step 1 Score Requirement:
No limits set
Minimum USMLE Step 2 Score Requirement:
No limits set
Attempts on any step: No limits set
CS required at time of application: Yes
including ECFMG certificate
USCE Requirement: Yes 2 different rotations 1
month each
Cut-Off time since graduation: No limits set but
must have any clinical experience in the last 2
years
Program offers couple match: Yes
Visas Sponsored or accepted: J1 visa

Virginia Commonwealth University Health System Obstetrics and Gynecology Residency Program

Specialty: Obstetrics and Gynecology
Program name: Virginia Commonwealth
University Health System Program
Program code: 220-51-11-299
NRMP Code: 1743220C0
Program type: University-based
State: Virginia

Address: VCU Health System
1250 E Marshall St, Richmond, VA 23298
Phone: (804) 828-8614
Fax: (804) 827-1229
Percentage of IMGs in the program: 0%
Minimum USMLE Step 1 Score Requirement: 203
Minimum USMLE Step 2 Score Requirement: 210
Attempts on any step: No limits set
CS required at time of application: Yes including ECFMG certificate
USCE Requirement: Yes 3 months within the last 4 years
Cut-Off time since graduation: 4 years
Program offers couple match: Yes
Visas Sponsored or accepted: J1 visa

Eastern Virginia Medical School Obstetrics and Gynecology Residency Program

Specialty: Obstetrics and Gynecology
Program name: Eastern Virginia Medical School Program
Program code: 220-51-21-298
NRMP Code: 2980220C0
Program type: Community-based
State: Virginia

Address: Eastern Virginia Medical School
825 Fairfax Ave, Norfolk, VA 23507
Phone: (757) 446-7470
Fax: (757) 446-7464
Percentage of IMGs in the program: 15%
Minimum USMLE Step 1 Score Requirement:
No limits set
Minimum USMLE Step 2 Score Requirement:
No limits set
Attempts on any step: Must pass on first
attempt
CS required at time of application: Yes
including ECFMG certificate
USCE Requirement: None
Cut-Off time since graduation: 8 years
Program offers couple match: Yes
Visas Sponsored or accepted: J1 visa

Carilion Clinic-Virginia Tech Carilion School of Medicine Obstetrics and Gynecology Residency Program

Specialty: Obstetrics and Gynecology
Program name: Carilion Clinic-Virginia Tech
Carilion School of Medicine Program
Program code: 220-51-31-300
NRMP Code: 1748220C0
Program type: Community-based university
affiliated hospital
State: Virginia

Address: Carilion Clinic Roanoke Memorial Hospital

1906 Belleview Ave SE, Roanoke, VA 24014

Phone: (540) 853-0427

Fax: (540) 983-1192

Percentage of IMGs in the program: 0%

Minimum USMLE Step 1 Score Requirement: No limits set

Minimum USMLE Step 2 Score Requirement: No limits set

Attempts on any step: Must pass on first attempt

CS required at time of application: No

USCE Requirement: None

Cut-Off time since graduation: No limits set

Program offers couple match: Yes

Visas Sponsored or accepted: J1 visa

Washington

University of Washington Obstetrics and Gynecology Residency Program

Specialty: Obstetrics and Gynecology

Program name: University of Washington Program
Program code: 220-54-21-301
NRMP Code: 1918220C0
Program type: University-based
State: Washington
Address: University of Washington School of Medicine
            1959 NE Pacific St, Seattle, WA 98195-6460
Phone: (206) 543-9626
Fax: (206) 543-3915
Percentage of IMGs in the program: 0%
Minimum USMLE Step 1 Score Requirement: No limits set
Minimum USMLE Step 2 Score Requirement: No limits set
Attempts on any step: Must pass on first attempt
CS required at time of application: No
USCE Requirement: None
Cut-Off time since graduation: No limits set
Program offers couple match: Yes
Visas Sponsored or accepted: J1 visa (H1b visa case by case)

West Virginia

Charleston Area Medical Center/West Virginia University (Charleston Division) Obstetrics and Gynecology Residency Program

Specialty: Obstetrics and Gynecology
Program name: Charleston Area Medical Center/West Virginia University (Charleston Division) Program
Program code: 220-55-11-303
NRMP Code: 1902220C0
Program type: Community-based university affiliated hospital
State: West Virginia
Address: West Virginia University Charleston Division

830 Pennsylvania Ave, Charleston, WV 25302
Phone: (304) 388-1515
Fax: (304) 388-1586
Percentage of IMGs in the program: 8% (Variable)
Minimum USMLE Step 1 Score Requirement: 200
Minimum USMLE Step 2 Score Requirement: 205
Attempts on any step: Must pass on first attempt
CS required at time of application: No
USCE Requirement: None

Cut-Off time since graduation: No limits set
Program offers couple match: Yes
Visas Sponsored or accepted: J1 visa

West Virginia University Obstetrics and Gynecology Residency Program

Specialty: Obstetrics and Gynecology
Program name: West Virginia University Program
Program code: 220-55-11-304
NRMP Code: 1837220C0
Program type: University-based
State: West Virginia
Address: West Virginia University Hospitals
One Medical Center Dr, Morgantown, WV 26506-9186
Phone: (304) 293-7542
Fax: (304) 293-5709
Percentage of IMGs in the program: 0%
Minimum USMLE Step 1 Score Requirement: No limits set
Minimum USMLE Step 2 Score Requirement: No limits set
Attempts on any step: Must pass on first attempt
CS required at time of application: No
USCE Requirement: None
Cut-Off time since graduation: No limits set

Program offers couple match: Yes
Visas Sponsored or accepted: J1 visa

Marshall University School of Medicine Obstetrics and Gynecology Residency Program

Specialty: Obstetrics and Gynecology
Program name: Marshall University School of Medicine Program
Program code: 220-55-21-344
NRMP Code: 3066220C0
Program type: Community-based university affiliated hospital
State: West Virginia
Address: Marshall University School of Medicine
        1600 Medical Center Dr, Huntington, WV 25701-3655
Phone: (304) 691-1454   Ext: 1454
Fax: (304) 691-1453
Percentage of IMGs in the program: 20%
Minimum USMLE Step 1 Score Requirement: 200 (188 previously)
Minimum USMLE Step 2 Score Requirement: 205 (196 previously)
Attempts on any step: No limits set
CS required at time of application: Yes
USCE Requirement: None
Cut-Off time since graduation: No limits set

Program offers couple match: Yes
Visas Sponsored or accepted: J1 visa

Wisconsin

Medical College of Wisconsin Affiliated Hospitals Obstetrics and Gynecology Residency Program

Specialty: Obstetrics and Gynecology
Program name: Medical College of Wisconsin Affiliated Hospitals Program
Program code: 220-56-31-307
NRMP Code: 1784220C0
Program type: University-based
State: Wisconsin
Address: Medical College of Wisconsin
9200 W Wisconsin Ave, Milwaukee, WI 53226
Phone: (414) 805-6658
Fax: (414) 805-6622
Percentage of IMGs in the program: 0%
Minimum USMLE Step 1 Score Requirement: No limits set
Minimum USMLE Step 2 Score Requirement: No limits set
Attempts on any step: No limits set

CS required at time of application: Yes including ECFMG certificate
USCE Requirement: None
Cut-Off time since graduation: No limits set
Program offers couple match: Yes
Visas Sponsored or accepted: J1 visa and H1b visa

University of Wisconsin Obstetrics and Gynecology Residency Program

Specialty: Obstetrics and Gynecology
Program name: University of Wisconsin Program
Program code: 220-56-21-306
NRMP Code: 1779220C0
Program type: University-based
State: Wisconsin
Address: Meriter Hospital
             202 S Park St, Madison, WI 53715
Phone: (608) 417-7358
Fax: (608) 417-1860
Percentage of IMGs in the program: 0%
Minimum USMLE Step 1 Score Requirement: No limits set
Minimum USMLE Step 2 Score Requirement: No limits set
Attempts on any step: Must pass on first attempt

CS required at time of application: Yes including ECFMG certificate
USCE Requirement: Yes
Cut-Off time since graduation: 5 years
Program offers couple match: Yes
Visas Sponsored or accepted: J1 visa

Aurora Health Care Obstetrics and Gynecology Residency Program

Specialty: Obstetrics and Gynecology
Program name: Aurora Health Care Program
Program code: 220-56-12-308
NRMP Code: 1787220C0
Program type: Community-based
State: Wisconsin
Address: Aurora Sinai Medical Center
            945 N 12th St, Milwaukee, WI 53201-0342
Phone: (414) 219-5725
Fax: (414) 219-5611
Percentage of IMGs in the program: 10%
Minimum USMLE Step 1 Score Requirement: No limits set
Minimum USMLE Step 2 Score Requirement: No limits set
Attempts on any step: Must pass on first attempt

CS required at time of application: Yes
including ECFMG certificate
USCE Requirement: Yes
Cut-Off time since graduation: 2 years
Program offers couple match: Yes
Visas Sponsored or accepted: No visa

I wish you good luck.

Thank you for buying our book.

Please, Please and Please take a minute to review our book on Amazon.

Match A Doc
Residency Guide

www.matchadoc.com